The Cleveland Clinic Guide to

OSTEOPOROSIS

Also in *The Cleveland Clinic Guide* Series

The Cleveland Clinic Guide to Arthritis

The Cleveland Clinic Guide to Diabetes

The Cleveland Clinic Guide to Fibromyalgia

The Cleveland Clinic Guide to Heart Attacks

The Cleveland Clinic Guide to Heart Failure

The Cleveland Clinic Guide to Infertility

The Cleveland Clinic Guide to Liver Disorders

The Cleveland Clinic Guide to Lung Cancer

The Cleveland Clinic Guide to Menopause

The Cleveland Clinic Guide to Pain Management

The Cleveland Clinic Guide to Prostate Cancer

The Cleveland Clinic Guide to Sleep Disorders

The Cleveland Clinic Guide to Speaking with Your Cardiologist

The Cleveland Clinic Guide to Thyroid Disorders

The Cleveland Clinic Guide to

OSTEOPOROSIS

Abby Abelson, MD

KAPLAN

PUBLISHING

New York

© 2010 Kaplan Publishing

Artwork by Joseph Kanasz, BFA. Reprinted with the permission of The Cleveland Clinic Center for Medical Art & Photograph © 2010.

Published by Kaplan Publishing, a division of Kaplan, Inc.
1 Liberty Plaza, 24th Floor
New York, NY 10006

Printed in the United States of America

10 9 8 7 6 5 4 3 2 1

Library of Congress Cataloging-in-Publication Data

Abelson, Abby.
   The Cleveland Clinic guide to osteoporosis / Abby Abelson.
     p. cm. — (Cleveland Clinic guide series)
   Includes bibliographical references and index.
   ISBN 978-1-60714-422-9 (alk. paper)
   1. Osteoporosis—Popular works. I. Cleveland Clinic Foundation.
II. Title. III. Title: Osteoporosis.
   RC931.O73A24 2010
   616.7'16—dc22

                               2009028596

Contents

Introduction

You rush to get off the plane, grab your luggage from the overhead baggage compartment, and suddenly feel an intense pain in your midback. You ignore it and continue with your fast-paced lifestyle. You think that it can't be anything serious, that you must have only pulled a muscle. After all, you live a healthy lifestyle, drink milk, and jog regularly.

The pain persists, so a few months later you go to the doctor. Your doctor gets an x-ray and diagnoses a compression fracture in your spine from osteoporosis.

Quickly, the truth hits: if this can happen to you—a young, active professional—it can happen to anyone. And it's true, osteoporosis and low bone mass are being diagnosed more often. But osteoporosis isn't a new disease.

Osteoporosis has existed since man began to walk the earth. Experts on aging believe that King David, who ruled Israel 3,000 years ago, may have suffered from the bone-depleting disease.

"My strength failed . . . and my bones are consumed," he wrote. "My bones wasted away through my anguished roaring all day long."

It was not until the 1820s that French pathologists coined the term *osteoporosis* to describe the porous state of certain bones they examined. More than a century would pass before the medical community could hone this rudimentary description into its current definition: a disease marked by a specific decrease in bone density and an increased risk of fractures.

Today, we are seeing osteoporosis and its precursor—low bone mass, or osteopenia—with increasing frequency as baby boomers near retirement. Currently, an astounding 28 million Americans have been diagnosed with varying degrees of low bone mass.

Yet many more people are unaware that their bone mass is slowly being depleted because they have no symptoms.

I recall getting a call from my own mother immediately after her hip fracture. I rushed over to see her. She was with the paramedics, lying on the floor of a bank after slipping in the February slush doing errands. She was unable to stand. It turned out that her hip was so badly shattered that she required hip replacement surgery the next day. Prior to this incident, we had no idea her bones were so fragile. Today, she is one of the lucky minority of hip fracture patients who retains her prefracture independence. Most patients are not as fortunate, as I witness daily through my work in

Cleveland Clinic's Center for Osteoporosis and Metabolic Bone Disease. Many have suffered painful fractures that have limited their independence and forced them to alter their lifestyles or move to a nursing home. For some, the disease has even resulted in death.

But osteoporosis and devastating fractures are not inevitable. Indeed, osteopenia and osteoporosis are both preventable *and* manageable. That's why I have written this Cleveland Clinic guide.

Education and early intervention are critical. It's important that we learn everything we can about maintaining bone health, which begins in childhood, throughout the course of our lives.

In this book, you will learn about osteoporosis and osteopenia. You will discover who is at risk, how they are diagnosed, and why bone thinning develops. You will read about current and promising treatments. Lastly, you will learn how to protect yourself and loved ones from falls and fractures.

As medical breakthroughs make it possible for us to live longer, it is absolutely essential that we try to maintain a healthy skeleton. Doing so will give us the freedom to remain active and enjoy those added years.

But it frequently takes commitment to changes in our daily habits to assure bone strength throughout life. It means adopting a more active lifestyle, including safe and appropriate exercise, starting when we are young. It means embracing a healthy, balanced diet—not only eating the right foods but also taking the right supplements.

Osteoporosis prevention also means regular checkups with your physician and bone density testing at appropriate intervals.

Intervening with bone-building medication when osteopenia or osteoporosis is diagnosed can prevent osteoporotic fractures in the hip, spine, and elsewhere—and avoid the need for troubling lifestyle adjustments.

Today, we are witness to a wealth of discoveries surrounding bone metabolism and the disorders that rob bones of their strength. These scientific gains have spurred development of a growing arsenal of medications, which allow us to prevent bone fragility and slow or even halt the progression of bone loss.

I have found it gratifying to see so many of my patients continue to lead active lives, without fractures, long after a diagnosis of osteoporosis. My hope is for a similarly strong and healthy future for us all.

Yours in good health,

Abby Abelson, MD
Interim Chair, Department of Rheumatic and
    Immunologic Diseases of the Orthopaedic &
    Rheumatologic Institute
Vice Chair for Education, Orthopaedic &
    Rheumatologic Institute
Education Director, Center for Osteoporosis and
    Metabolic Bone Disease

Chapter 1

Bones: The Framework of Our Lives

Truthfully, most of us pay little attention to our skeletal health until we break a bone. Just ask someone who's fractured a forearm and can't write or use the computer. Or can't walk or drive because he's broken an ankle. Or needs help dressing and toileting because of a fractured hip.

It is at these times that our body's architectural framework comes into sharp focus. Suddenly it's clear that without our bones, we'd be little more than shapeless forms, unable to move or bear weight. Our bones act as levers that allow muscles and tendons to extend and contract—to lift, carry, and propel us. As we move, the long bones in our arms and legs absorb and distribute the physical impact.

Our bones also serve as a pharmacy, storing minerals such as calcium and phosphorus and then dispensing them into the bloodstream, where they travel to cells and muscles throughout the body.

The skeleton plays a vital role, too, in safeguarding our organs. The skull protects the brain. (Hold a newborn and you'll notice the "soft spot" on top of the baby's head where the skull bones are still knitting together.) Our vertebrae encircle the spinal cord. Our ribs cradle our heart and lungs.

Our skeletons are surprisingly light because of the way our bones are structured. Researchers David B. Burr and Charles H. Turner compare fully developed bones to corrugated cardboard, with a hard outer layer protecting an inner spongy core. Most bones in our body are constructed with both these types of tissue: cortical bone and trabecular bone.

• • • *Fast Fact* • • •

Cortical bone is dense and compact. This outer bony layer provides mechanical strength, bears most of our weight, and gives shape to our skeleton. Cortical bone represents 80 percent of our total bone mass.

Trabecular bone is porous and sponge like and contains the marrow. It runs through the middle of long bones, is found at their ends, makes up the bulk of our vertebrae—the bones that make up our spinal column—and resides within large, flat bones such as those in the pelvis. Trabecular bone represents 20 percent of our bone mass. It is the type of bone that may be initially vulnerable to osteoporosis.

• • •

A View of Bone's "Microarchitecture"

Bone loss begins with deterioration in the microarchitecture of the skeleton. To understand how this occurs, it's useful to look through the microscope to see how bone—a living, growing tissue—behaves.

Bones are made up of tiny, hard mineral crystals bound to a matrix, or soft framework, of collagen. Collagen is made up of long, thin, intertwined protein chains. Our remarkable bodies combine just the right amounts of minerals for strength and collagen for resilience to absorb the impact of walking, running, and other stresses.

During childhood and adolescence, bones are created—or sculpted—through a dynamic, constant process called bone modeling. Young bones slowly shift position as they grow. New bone forms on top of existing bone tissue at one site. At the same time, old bone tissue is removed from other sites.

• • • *Fast Fact* • • •

Boys see the most significant growth in bone mass between ages 13 and 17. Bone continues to build up in their lower spines and thigh bones until about age 20. For both sexes, bone mass tends to peak in the early 20s.

• • •

Forming new bone is the job of special "builder" cells called osteoblasts. But they are just half of the equation. Osteoblasts work in concert with special bone "carver" cells called osteoclasts. Osteoclasts break down old bone by dissolving minerals, a process called resorption.

Imagine a construction crew building a road. The osteoclasts are like jackhammer operators, carving holes in old pavement to clear the way for other crew members to lay down a scaffolding, then fill it with concrete, layer by layer, until it sets and hardens. Similarly, the mineral-rich collagen scaffolding in bone, applied in orderly layers, hardens into tough, resilient bone.

As children and adolescents experience skeletal growth, the osteoblasts are dominant—building ever greater bone mass, density, and strength. Large amounts of bone are formed and resorbed during this time.

After age 20, skeletal growth slows and then stops. Bone no longer builds up at new sites on existing bone. However, bone modeling continues throughout our lives for healing purposes. New bone is formed when needed to bridge a fracture, repair small cracks, or smooth deformities.

Red Flag

Bone begins as cartilage in the fetus. During childhood and adolescence, bone size, strength, and density increase by leaps and bounds. Young females or males in the grip of eating disorders such as anorexia nervosa or bulimia nervosa sidestep the natural buildup of bone during childhood and adolescence and are at great risk for experiencing early and significant bone loss. If you have ever suffered from an eating disorder, ask your doctor if he or she recommends a bone density test to evaluate your skeletal health.

The dynamic process of bone buildup and bone breakdown continues as well, albeit through a different process—bone "remodeling." Rather than bone forming at new sites, existing bone is continuously dissolved, or resorbed, and replenished.

Our bodies must orchestrate a delicate balance between osteoclast and osteoblast activity to maintain the bone mass that we have until we reach skeletal maturity, during our third decade.

The cycle of replacing old bone with new maintains the skeleton's mechanical and structural integrity. In this way, adult bone is entirely replaced approximately every ten years, according to the U.S. Surgeon General.

The stages of the remodeling cycle can vary. Bone resorption may last only a few weeks. Bone formation, however, is slower and can take up to four months. In healthy individuals, bone resorption and formation are well synchronized.

Osteoporosis and Bone Loss

When bone remodeling is imbalanced—when bone resorption speeds ahead of bone replacement or when bone formation lags behind bone resorption—the net result is reduced bone mass. Primary osteoporosis happens because at some point, we begin to lose more bone mass than we gain due to faulty bone remodeling.

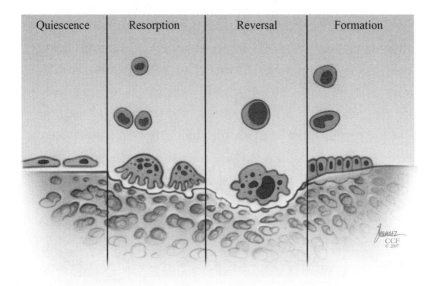

| Quiescence | Resorption | Reversal | Formation |

Bone is constantly being remodeled. Osteoclasts resorb small areas of bone which are then filled in by the action of osteoblasts.

Why Do I Hear Bone Loss Referred to in Bank Account Terms?

The skeleton is sometimes compared to a bank, where calcium and phosphorus "deposits" and "withdrawals" are made. With regular deposits during childhood and adolescence, our bones become larger, heavier, and denser as new bone is added to the skeleton. For most of us, the pace of bone formation exceeds the pace of bone resorption until our third decade. However, for some of us, withdrawals can begin to exceed deposits as early as age 20.

It's true that heredity helps to determine our bone mass. But our bones also need a good supply of calcium and phosphorus for normal everyday activity. We can accomplish this easily by

- eating a diet rich in calcium and vitamin D;
- taking vitamin and mineral supplements;
- getting regular weight-bearing exercise to stimulate bone formation; and
- avoiding tobacco and excessive alcohol use.

How Does Bone "Theft" Occur?

When we are not taking in enough essential minerals and vitamins, regulatory mechanisms enable the body to take minerals from our bones to supply the body's needs. Calcium that is "banked" in our bones may be needed for careful regulation of the calcium level in the blood. For example, an expectant mother contributes calcium from her own bones to supply her growing fetus, but in most cases, the body beautifully makes up for this in the postpartum period. For teenage mothers, however, whose skeletal systems may not have matured, this process of resorption can leave their bone accounts depleted.

Bone resorption can also accompany changes in the levels of regulating hormones and vitamin D. Estrogen, testosterone, parathyroid hormone, and calcitonin are all hormones that regulate the activity of osteoclasts and osteoblasts. Their goal: to maintain the right balance of minerals and protein (too much mineral, and our bones become brittle; too much protein, and they become soft).

How Does Estrogen Affect Bone Health?

As we will discuss in more detail throughout this book, estrogen helps maintain bone mass in men as well as in women. Estrogen deficiency accelerates the rate of bone turnover, tilting the delicate balance of bone formation and resorption. Bones grow thin and more porous—particularly the trabecular bone in the spine, which is a common place for an asymptomatic fracture. Other common sites of fractures from osteoporosis are the wrist and hips, but any bone can fracture from osteoporosis.

Estrogen levels in our system can fall for a variety of reasons:

- **Age.** Both men and women experience bone loss after age 50, but men experience more rapid bone loss after age 60.

- **Menopause.** Most women experience their most significant bone loss somewhere between the ages of 50 and 57—at menopause when estrogen production decreases and then virtually stops.

- **Anorexia.** Eating disorders, such as anorexia or bulimia, and very low-calorie diets are associated with low bone density and osteoporosis. In addition, overexercising may cause estrogen levels to fall and periods to lapse. When low body weight and excess exercise lead to the cessation of menstrual periods in women, there is a high risk of osteoporosis.

How Can Diet Affect My Risk of Bone Loss?

Calcium and phosphorus are considered key factors in bone health and bone loss. Calcium is the major building block of bone, so calcium intake remains important throughout our lives. Unfortunately, elderly bodies often are less efficient at absorbing calcium and vitamin D. In addition, according to the World Health Organization, the older we get, the fewer dairy products we tend to consume.

We know that getting adequate calcium and vitamin D is important for growing bones and for maintaining bone mass. Increasingly, research points to the profound importance of vitamin D. Vitamin D helps us absorb calcium. Vitamin D insufficiency has been shown to lead to fractures from osteoporosis and to muscle weakness, which can result in an increased risk for falls. People get vitamin D from their diet, dietary supplements, and exposure to sunlight. Sun exposure allows ultraviolet radiation to penetrate the skin and convert a substance in the skin to active vitamin D3.

Is It True That Carbonated Drinks Negatively Affect Bone Health?

Carbonated beverages are now a dietary staple in the form of soda, sparkling water, and energy drinks. But the phosphate additives they contain may negatively impact bone health in two ways:

1. Young people who choose to drink these beverages *instead of* milk are depriving themselves of the calcium that can help them achieve peak bone mass.

2. While no evidence confirms that high phosphate consumption accelerates bone loss, high phosphate intake does increase parathyroid hormone (PTH) secretion. As we've read, PTH is one of the hormones that regulates calcium levels in our bones.

In addition, excess PTH is the culprit in hyperpara-thyroidism, a condition associated with bone resorption and secondary osteoporosis.

Is It True That Steroids Can Trigger Bone Resorption?

If you have severe asthma, inflammatory bowel disease, or a rheumatic or immune disorder or you are a transplant recipient, chances are you've been on prednisone or another corticosteroid. Taking corticosteroids for extended periods can cause osteoporosis in three ways:

1. Steroids interfere with the body's ability to absorb calcium.
2. Steroids cause extra calcium to be excreted through the urine.
3. Steroids have a direct, negative impact on bone cells.

Does My Level of Physical Activity Affect My Bone Health?

Exercise is a vital component of healthy living, but weight-bearing exercise is particularly important in our increasingly sedentary world. By bearing the weight of our bodies when we exercise, we stimulate bone formation and help to counter bone resorption. Studies show that astronauts who exercise vigorously in space still lose bone mass because they are exercising under weightless conditions. Gravity adds to the many benefits of such "earthbound" exercises as jogging, aerobics, skating, and weight lifting.

Is It Possible to Rebuild Bone Mass?

That is just what osteoporosis experts hope will happen with currently available medications, as well as promising new treatments. Once the bones become thinned and osteopenia develops, osteoporosis may not be far off. As the precursor to osteoporosis, osteopenia sends up a red flag for doctors to begin treatment that will stem the tide of bone loss.

Today, physicians have an arsenal of medications to choose from to help build up bone strength. Working directly on bone cells, new antiresorptive agents may be able to slow bone breakdown by osteoclasts. According to the U.S. Surgeon General, studies suggest that even a 10 percent increase in peak bone mass could decrease risks of hip fractures among Caucasian women by 30 percent.

As medical science discovers ways to help us live longer and healthier lives, it is important that we maintain strong skeletons to enable us to remain active throughout our elderly years. Cardiologists have discovered strategies to maintain heart health, and we see many individuals actively playing tennis, running, and skiing into their 80s. Only by addressing bone health can we hope to maintain bones that are strong enough to support these enjoyable activites. When I see an otherwise completely healthy patient who falls on the tennis court and fractures her hip in her 70s, I am so distressed knowing that earlier attention to her bones could have prevented this devastating fracture.

Now that you know a little bit about bone health issues, let's take a look at what osteoporosis actually is.

Chapter 2

What Is Osteoporosis?

Many people don't discover that they have osteoporosis until they suffer their first fracture. For some, the triggering event can be as innocent as a sneeze, a step off the curb, or an overly enthusiastic hug.

Translated literally, *osteoporosis* means "porous bones." Our skeletons act as a storehouse for calcium and the other minerals that strengthen the 200 bones in our body. Strong bones hold us upright, protect our organs, and keep us mobile. But when minerals leach from the bones, they become brittle, weak, and ripe for fracture.

The National Institutes of Health defines *osteoporosis* as "a disease characterized by low bone mass and structural deterioration of bone tissue, leading to bone fragility and an increased risk of fractures."

Other Bone Diseases

Your doctor must confirm a correct diagnosis in order to recommend the most appropriate treatment for your low bone density, osteopenia, or osteoporosis. Your physician will evaluate your bone density and your fracture risk and evaluate your medical history to determine whether other medical conditions affecting bone are present. Other bone diseases can cause fractures as well, and it is important to have a full evaluation to determine whether another condition is present that can cause bone loss. Some of these additional conditions include the following:

- **Hyperparathyroidism.** An endocrine disorder that weakens the bones as overactive parathyroid glands secrete too much hormone, triggering calcium withdrawals from bone

- **Osteomalacia.** A nutritional disorder that softens the bones due to insufficient levels of vitamin D, phosphorus, or calcium

- **Paget's disease.** A rheumatologic condition that usually targets middle-aged and elderly individuals, primarily men, increasing their rate of bone resorption. The replacement bone is not well-organized, leading to pain and bone deformity.

Any bone in any part of the body can break as a result of osteoporosis. More than 50 percent of the fractures attributed to osteoporosis each year involve the bones of the spine (vertebrae). There may be no symptoms other than a loss of height or some back pain. However, in severe cases, so many vertebrae fracture that the spine collapses forward, constricting both abdominal organs and lungs and making breathing difficult.

Nearly 25 percent of osteoporotic fractures affect the lower arm or wrist. Though osteoporosis is typically thought of as an "old woman's disease," these types of fractures more often happen in people who are in their 50s, like Kate.

Kate

Kate was sailing through her early 50s, the picture of health, when she slipped on the ice and severely fractured her wrist. Her physician knew that wrist fractures that occur after a fall from standing height are most probably related to osteoporosis, so she suggested that Kate have a bone mineral density (BMD) test for osteoporosis. A few days later, the doctor called her with the news: the tests confirmed that Kate had osteoporosis. She was devastated.

"I have osteoporosis. I can't believe it," she told a friend she met for lunch. "I'm only 52! My mother in her nursing home, maybe, but not me!" But Kate was further surprised to hear that her 49-year-old friend DeeDee had also recently been given a BMD test. "My doctor said that I don't have osteoporosis, but I'm mighty close," DeeDee confided. She explained that her doctor had her start taking weekly medication and calcium and vitamin D supplements to build up her bones. DeeDee also started weight training and, at the urging of her doctor, had quit smoking. Kate was relieved to discover that there were immediate, simple lifestyle changes she could make to protect herself from further bone loss and injury, and she was surprised to find that so many women her age had similar problems.

"You know, I would have kept right on going if I hadn't fractured my wrist. I never had any symptoms at all," Kate said. This is true for many patients whose first indication of a problem is a lower arm or wrist fracture.

Another 25 percent of fractures involve the hip. Hip fractures primarily affect the elderly and are the most ominous. Statistics show that about 20 percent of patients die within a year of fracturing a hip; the odds of survival plummet with advancing age, and the outlook is bleaker for men than for women. Men are twice as likely to die in the hospital after a hip fracture, and 31 percent of men will die in the first year following a hip fracture.

Is Osteoporosis a Common Disease?

How common is this stealthy, bone-depleting disease? Consider these statistics:

- Osteoporosis is our country's most common skeletal disorder; more than 44 million Americans are at risk for it.

- Approximately 10 million Americans already have osteoporosis—8 million women and 2 million men.

- Thirty-four million more of us have osteopenia (low bone density or low bone mass), which can lead to osteoporosis if left untreated.

- After age 50, one in two women and one in eight men will suffer an osteoporosis-related fracture. This adds up to more than 1.5 million bone fractures due to osteoporosis every year.

What Are the Key Risk Factors?

Many conditions can place someone at risk for osteoporosis. Some of these risk factors are being female, being over age 50, having a slender build, and having a family history of fractures or falls.

Being Female. Eighty percent of those affected by osteoporosis are women, but bone density gradually diminishes in both sexes after peak bone mass is achieved. In men, that happens around age 30; in women, it happens around age 35. However, men start off with higher bone mass and have the advantage of larger, stronger bones. After turning 30, men lose about 4 percent of their bone mass per decade. Women, on the other hand, get hit with a double whammy. Around menopause, their supply of estrogen, a female hormone that helps maintain bone mass, dwindles. Bone loss rapidly accelerates; after menopause, women lose an alarming 15 percent of their bone mass per decade. With more women choosing to forgo hormone replacement therapy, which protects against bone thinning after menopause, osteoporosis poses an even greater threat. Finally, women live longer and represent a larger proportion of the elderly.

Being Older Than 50. As we age, the risk of osteoporosis increases for both men and women. Calcium is the building block of bones. As we age, more and more calcium "withdrawals" are made, and our bone mineral density declines. And our population is aging. By 2010, an estimated 12 million Americans over 50 are expected to have osteoporosis; by 2020, that number is projected to rise to 14 million. By 2010,

40 million Americans are expected to develop osteopenia; by 2020, 47 million cases of osteopenia are anticipated.

Having a Slight Build. Those who start off with relatively low bone density are at higher risk for osteoporosis due to the body's constant formation and "resorption" of bone. Bone is living, dynamic tissue—like hair, skin, and nails—which constantly replenishes itself through a complex process involving teamwork by osteoblasts and osteoclasts. A host of hormones, including growth hormone and sex hormones such as estrogen and testosterone, provide the fuel for these cells. Patients who have low body weight may have lower bone density due to several factors. Body weight alone may contribute to the mechanical loading of bone that helps maintain and increase bone density. There may be conversion of adrenal androgens to estrogens in some patients with a higher percentage of adipose (fat) tissue. In addition, very thin people are more likely to fracture if they fall, since they have less padding to protect their bones. For all these reasons and more, low body weight is associated with increased bone fracture rates at many skeletal sites, including the hips and vertebrae.

Family History or Ethnicity. Family history and ethnicity do contribute to risks. If there is osteoporosis in your family, then you may be genetically predisposed to develop the same condition. And if you are a Caucasian, Asian, or Hispanic woman, your risks for osteoporosis are greater than if you are an African American woman. However, recent studies have shown that many dark-skinned women, such as African American women, have a unique risk factor: because their skin takes a longer period of sun exposure to produce vitamin D, their levels of this critical vitamin may be abnormally low. This would put them at a greater risk of osteoporosis than previously considered. Moreover, many ethnic groups have a higher incidence of lactose intolerance, so avoiding dairy products may lead to inadequate dietary calcium, putting them at risk for osteoporosis as well.

"Low Risk" Is Not the Same as "No Risk"

When we think of osteoporosis, it's easy to picture the elderly woman with the dowager's hump. True, being female, over 50, and Caucasian should raise a red flag. But being male, young, or African American doesn't necessarily let you off the hook. Osteoporosis is a disease that cuts across gender, age, and ethnicity; those less likely to develop osteoporosis still face *some* risk.

Just ask Jack, age 72. What man thinks he could be at risk for what many wrongly believe is a woman's disease? Like Kate, Jack's discovery that he had osteoporosis was purely accidental. One day on the golf course, he simply bent down to tuck his tee into the green. The pain in his back was agonizing. Jack sought immediate medical attention. After x-raying Jack's spine, his doctor diagnosed a vertebral fracture and ordered a BMD test, which confirmed that Jack had osteoporosis.

At the other end of the spectrum is Holly, an extremely thin, underdeveloped 14-year-old. She eats very little, runs five miles a day, and weighs herself religiously to make sure she hasn't gained an ounce. She menstruates only four or five times per year. Holly doesn't know it, but her eating disorder, anorexia nervosa, will put her at high risk of osteopenia (low bone mass) by the time she is just 28 years old. Denying herself calcium-rich foods, limiting food intake, and exercising obsessively during adolescence are depleting her bone mass just when it should be gaining strength.

A Large Price Tag

In 2004, the U.S. Surgeon General's office produced a sobering report on the state of America's bone health. The news was not good. By the year 2020, half of all Americans 50 and over could be at risk of fractures from osteoporosis or osteopenia if significant progress is not made. By the year 2040, the number of hip fractures could double or triple.

In 2005, osteoporosis-related fractures were responsible for an estimated $19 billion in costs. By 2025, experts predict that the costs of treating osteoposis in America will rise to $25.3 billion.

In 2002, the National Osteoporosis Foundation released the following statistics:

- In 2002, hip fractures alone cost $18 billion.

- Each hip fracture cost between $30,100 and $43,400.

- Overall lifetime costs of a single hip fracture were projected at well over $80,000 (in 2002 dollars).

Hospital care alone consumes half the direct costs of fractures from osteoporosis; secondary nursing home care consumes the rest. While healthcare costs are picked up at first by insurance, Medicare, or Medicaid, these same costs are borne by society as a whole and will continue to rise.

For the individual with osteoporosis, fractures also come at tremendous personal cost: loss of productivity, forced change in lifestyle, and loss of self-esteem. Two-thirds of patients with hip fractures may never return to their prior level of functioning. Many require nursing home care or additional care.

Best of Times, Worst of Times

To borrow a famous line from Charles Dickens's *A Tale of Two Cities,* it is now the best of times and the worst of times for osteoporosis. In the past two decades, we have learned more about this disease than ever before. More tests are available today than in the past, and more medications to stem the tide of bone loss, build bone density, and reduce the risk of future fractures. Risk factors for osteoporosis have been identified by the scientific community, and they have commanded media attention.

Yet most of those at risk for, or suffering from, osteoporosis-related fractures are not properly diagnosed or treated, because current knowledge has not been applied, because of lack of access to medical care, or because treatment recommendations are ignored. Even after a fracture, most people are not appropriately evaluated for osteoporosis. And in many cases, patients who are diagnosed and treated do not stay on their prescribed medications.

Osteoporosis is the "silent disease," not only because of its lack of symptoms but also because few people think to talk about it with family, friends, or, most importantly, their physicians. It rarely makes the list of complaints that spur a doctor's visit.

How Has Such a Huge Threat to Our Health Remained So Undercover?

Some problems are easy to ignore. Imagine the busy female executive, traveling for business, who reaches for luggage from the overhead rack. Suddenly, she feels a pain in the middle of her back under her bra line. She thinks she's strained a muscle.

It's easy to ignore minor pain in these circumstances. Months can pass, and the fracture goes undetected until the woman sees her doctor for a routine problem, such as a nagging cough. The physician orders a chest x-ray and says, "You've got a fracture in your lower thoracic spine." A BMD test is ordered. She, like millions of others, is shocked to learn that osteoporosis has been quietly sapping her bones of their strength.

Perhaps because the specter of heart attack and cancer loom so large in our society, physicians as well as patients may pay more attention to symptoms such as chest pain, high cholesterol, and abdominal pain. While we mustn't diminish the importance of those health concerns, the fact is that osteoporosis remains underdiagnosed and undertreated.

In 2004, Surgeon General Richard H. Carmona estimated that the number of men with osteoporosis was probably four times higher and the number of women nearly three times higher than reported. Much of what can be done to lessen the burden of osteoporosis is ignored, he added, urging healthcare providers, policy makers, and families to right this wrong. For example, even when osteoporosis is diagnosed, many patients who require medication and monitoring lack prescription coverage or cannot access needed medical care.

In addition, studies indicate that one year after starting medication for osteoporosis, only 40 to 60 percent of patients still take their medicine as prescribed.

Finally, relatively few inroads have been made into reducing the negative effects of smoking, alcohol, poor diet, and lack of exercise on bone health.

So the news is both good and bad. While medical science has made progress in the diagnosis and treatment of osteoporosis, great challenges remain to ensure that patients are appropriately evaluated, treated, and followed.

What Is Being Done to Increase Awareness and Treatment Options for Osteoporosis?

The National Osteoporosis Foundation and many other healthcare groups are adopting a strong advocacy role to encourage increased research into, education on, and early diagnosis of osteoporosis. Past advocacy efforts succeeded in standardizing reimbursement for BMD tests for Medicare patients who are at risk of osteoporosis. But more needs to be done—in terms of overall health, a woman's risk of hip fracture is equal to her *combined* risks of breast, uterine, and ovarian cancer.

It is said that osteoporosis is a "pediatric disease with adult manifestations." Children and young adults need adequate calcium, vitamin D, and exercise to build up bone strength so that they achieve their best potential peak bone mass, as

You Can Help

To become an advocate for osteoporosis awareness and research, individuals can write letters to and email their elected officials, urging them to support legislation and funding for osteoporosis research; bone density testing; and the care of patients with osteoporosis, including appropriate medications.

they should, in their early 20s. Unfortunately, recent data suggest that children and adolescents are not getting sufficient calcium, vitamin D, or exercise. The couch potato habits of television watching and hours on the computer have become prevalent, and soda products have taken over from milk as the preferred drink for many young people.

Early education is vital, and school gym classes are an ideal place for teachers to discuss the importance of bone health and weight-bearing exercise along with weight management. Unfortunately, gym classes are rapidly disappearing due to school budget cuts. The same financial constraints prevent registered dietitians from working with schools to get calcium-rich foods into the cafeteria and teaching students about the importance of healthy food choices.

However, the U.S. Department of Health and Human Services' Office on Women's Health, the Centers for Disease Control and Prevention, and the National Osteoporosis Foundation are doing their part. The groups joined forces to launch the National Bone Health Campaign, targeted at 9- to 12-year-old girls. After researching the best way to share

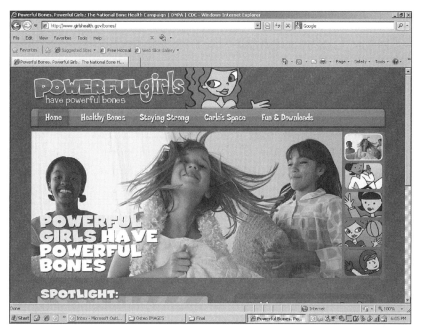

This "Powerful Girls" website is an example of public education that promotes bone health.

information with this age group, the campaign adopted the slogan "Powerful Girls Have Powerful Bones" and launched an interactive website: *www.girlshealth.gov/bones/*. Quizzes and games help to educate preadolescent girls about the importance of diet, weight-bearing exercise, and calcium intake on their bone health.

There have, unfortunately, been recent threats to patient access to bone density testing due to cuts in reimbursement for these tests. Without access to this test, most Americans would not be able to get evaluation of their bone health or get treatment for their osteopenia and osteoporosis. Recent legislation has been presented to address this important public health issue in both the Senate and the House as the

How Bone Density Is Measured

The most common way to measure bone density is a DXA bone density test, which utilizes x-rays to measure bone mineral density. The test is safe and involves lying on your back under a scanner machine for 10–15 minutes. The results allow your bone density to be compared to that of other individuals your age, as well as young healthy adults. The data can be used to predict the risk of future fracture, as well as the need for treatment.

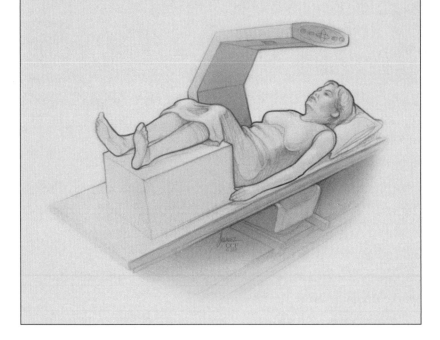

Medicare Fracture Prevention and Osteoporosis Testing Act of 2009 (S. 769/H.R. 1894). If passed, this bill will secure Medicare reimbursement funding for bone density testing and authorize a study of how reduced reimbursement affects patients.

• • • *Fast Fact* • • •

You can find information about government advocacy
at the National Osteoporosis Foundation's website:
www.nof.org/advocacy/.

• • •

It's Never Too Late

As the Surgeon General Richard H. Carmona said when the
2004 report was released, "Osteoporosis isn't just your grandmother's disease. We all need to take better care of our bones.
The good news is that you are never too old or too young to
improve your bone health.

"With healthy nutrition, physical activity every day, and
regular medical checkups and screenings, Americans of all
ages can have strong bones and live longer, healthier lives.
Likewise, if it's diagnosed in time, osteoporosis can be treated
with new drugs that help prevent bone loss and rebuild bone
before life-threatening fractures occur."

In upcoming chapters of this book, we will provide you
with information on the root causes of osteoporosis; your risks
for osteoporosis and fracture; preventive measures, including
how to get the correct diagnosis; treatment for men as well
as for women; and creating a prevention plan that includes
making your home safe.

The end result will be a healthier you.

Chapter 3

Are You at Risk?

In chapter 2 we met Kate: she is female, over 50, and Caucasian. The severity of her wrist fracture tipped her doctor off to the possibility of osteoporosis. But suppose she had other risk factors that might have helped her be more aware of her chances of developing osteoporosis? A slender frame. A mother who had suffered a hip fracture in her 70s. A 20-year history of smoking, which started in her late teens.

With that abundance of risk factors, a diagnosis of osteoporosis is hard to miss. But what about people we would *never* suspect of being at risk for osteoporosis—perhaps someone like you?

You're healthy, or so you think. You get up, start your day with a cup of coffee, head to work, and run errands on your lunch hour. When you do grab something to eat, it's usually filling but still something you know isn't the best for you—say, from the fast-food restaurant just down the street.

You whip back into work and sit for the rest of the day in your office, hunched over computer reports with the phone beneath your chin. You feel healthy, you look fit, and you're active. Everyone is always amazed at how much energy you have. But when you go in for your annual physical, your doctor decides it's time for a bone screening for osteoporosis.

"I'm only forty-five!" you sputter. "Aren't you supposed to start screening for that at fifty?"

"Yes, that's normally the way it goes," your doctor replies. "But I attended an interesting seminar last week, and, you know, sometimes they *can* teach an old doctor new tricks. Did you know that the surgeon general's report on bone health says that by 2020, one in two Americans over fifty will be at risk for fractures from osteoporosis? You have at least one risk factor: you went into menopause early, at age forty-three . . . and didn't your mother have a hip fracture?"

A bone density test is painless, takes hardly any time, and will give your doctor a good snapshot of where you stand right now. If there is a problem, you can take preventive steps immediately. Don't you think that's better than waiting five more years and hoping you aren't losing bone mass?

Osteoporosis Risk Factors

The major risk factors for osteoporosis, according to the National Osteoporosis Foundation, are as follows:

- **Age.** Risks increase with advancing age for both men and women.

- **Gender.** Women start with less bone tissue than men and experience dramatic bone loss after menopause.

- **Fracture history.** A personal or family history of adult fractures, especially of the spine, increases risks.

- **Ethnicity.** Caucasian and Asian women are at higher risk (though risks for Hispanic and African American women are still significant).

- **Build.** A slight build and weight under 127 pounds will increase risks of osteoporosis.

- **Estrogen deficiency.** Women whose periods stop before age 48 or who have undergone menopause face higher risks.

- **Lifestyle.** Less-than-healthy habits, such as smoking, excess drinking, avoiding exercise, and not getting enough calcium, will hasten bone loss.

- **Medications or chronic illnesses.** Health problems and their treatment can reduce bone mass.

Can Medications or Surgeries Increase My Risk of Bone Loss?

Sometimes, the very medicines we need to manage a medical condition can also deplete bone mass. Say you undergo a life-saving organ transplantation. It's a given that you will be on lifelong medication to prevent your immune system from rejecting your new organ. But immune-suppressing drugs may reduce bone density. So it's important to talk with your doctor about regular BMD testing.

Here are some other medications, which, while effective, increase our risks for osteoporosis:

- **Glucocorticoids (corticosteroids).** Used to control inflammation in conditions ranging from asthma to rheumatoid arthritis.

- **Anticonvulsants.** Used to control seizure disorders.

- **Heparin.** This blood thinner is used to prevent clotting.

- **Gonadotropin-releasing hormone (GnRH) agonists.** Used to treat endometriosis and fibroids in women and prostate cancer in men.

- **Chemotherapy, certain cytotoxic drugs such as methotrexate, and aromitase inhibitors.** Used to combat cancer.

- **Aluminum-containing antacids.** Used to heal peptic ulcers.

- **Thyroid hormone replacement therapy.** Used to boost an underactive thyroid gland when prescribed in excessive doses.

Some surgical procedures used to correct serious health problems also raise our risks of osteoporosis. For example, when the stomach is severely damaged by a peptic ulcer, the diseased portion may have to be removed in a procedure called a gastrectomy. While absolutely necessary, the operation interferes with the ability to absorb bone-building nutrients. Thus, patients face a higher likelihood of osteoporosis in their future.

Similarly, gastric bypass surgery has become an increasingly popular solution for overweight Americans who want to reduce the many health risks of obesity. Yet the long-term impact of bypassing portions of the intestine during these surgeries is unknown. One study has shown that bone mineral density decreases the first year after gastric bypass surgery and that patients no longer absorb the recommended daily allowances of calcium and vitamin D without supplementation.

Can Other Illnesses Cause Osteoporosis Onset?

We are all dealt certain cards at birth. We can't do anything about our gender, ethnicity, bone structure, or family history. And there is no sidestepping the need for medical therapy that saves our lives or makes them livable, despite risks of osteoporosis. We may have to live with medical conditions that in and of themselves trigger bone loss, such as the following:

- **Endocrine disorders, which alter hormone production.** These include type 1 diabetes, hyperthyroidism, Cushing's syndrome, primary or secondary hypogonadism, and hyperprolactinemia. Primary hyperparathyroidism, a condition that results from an overproduction of parathyroid hormone by the parathyroid glands, can result in osteoporosis. Eating and nutritional disorders, such as anorexia nervosa, also fall into this category.

- **Gastrointestinal (digestive) disorders, which interfere with nutrient absorption.** These include inflammatory bowel disease, malabsorption syndrome, and severe liver disease.

- **Bone marrow disorders.** These include multiple myeloma, lymphoma, leukemia, hemophilia, mastocytosis, and hemochromatosis.

- **Genetic syndromes that affect the skeleton.** These include osteogenesis imperfecta and hypophosphatasia.

In addition, chronic conditions, such as multiple sclerosis, rheumatoid arthritis, chronic obstructive pulmonary disease (COPD), and chronic renal failure, can increase our risks of osteoporosis. But appreciating those risks and working in partnership with our physicians to manage our conditions can help us maintain healthy bones.

Say that you have type 1 diabetes. The best way to care for yourself is to control your blood sugar. Regularly monitor your blood glucose levels, and you'll prevent diabetic complications down the road. If you add bone density monitoring to that preventive strategy, then you'll ensure that any bone loss is detected and treated.

Can I Do Anything to Reduce My Risk of Developing Osteoporosis?

As noted earlier, some of the major risk factors of osteoporosis simply cannot be avoided, such as age, family history, gender, or ethnicity. But even when your risks cannot be altered, adopting healthy lifestyle measures, such as committing to a weight-bearing exercise program, can boost your bone health.

And it's never too late to reap the benefits of quitting cigarettes and limiting alcohol intake. Smoking hampers the skeleton's ability to absorb calcium and vitamin D. Smokers generally weigh less and are less physically active, so their risks of fracture are higher.

Alcohol interferes with vitamin D absorption and bone formation and may increase the loss of bone-building calcium and magnesium. Chronic alcohol intake of more than two drinks per day has been reported to result in osteopenia or osteoporosis.

Excessive drinking also increases our risks of falls and, therefore, fractures.

Other factors that make us susceptible to falls and fractures include these:

- Impaired vision
- Dementia
- Poor health
- A history of recent falls

Being Proactive

The bottom line: Know your risks. Address any factors—diet, activity level, or other lifestyle habits—that will help to preserve your bone health. If you have to live with some risks because caring for a health condition demands it, then work with your doctor to monitor your bone density.

Experts recommend bone mineral density testing for

- all women age 65 and over;
- all postmenopausal women under age 65 with one or more risk factors for osteoporosis;

- all patients—male and female—who have suffered a "fragility" fracture; and

- all men age 70 and older.

Note that insurance may not pay for bone mineral density tests before age 65. But BMD testing is important to determine if there is low bone mass so that it can be treated early if appropriate.

Now that you are aware of the conditions that may place you at risk of having low bone density or osteoporosis, you can speak with your physician about whether a DXA is appropriate, either as an initial assessment or as follow-up from your previous test. In addition, you can change your habits to modify the risks that you can change, like calcium intake, Vitamin D intake, exercise, smoking, and drinking alcohol. While we cannot control our genetic predisposition to osteoporosis or stop using medications like prednisone, which may be indicated for treatment of other medical illnesses, we can reduce our risk factors for osteoporosis on our road to bone health.

Chapter 4

Men: The Hidden Minority

True, osteoporosis affects fewer men than women. But some 1.5 million men over age 65 have osteoporosis. And another 3.5 million are at risk—particularly Caucasian men like Jack.

Jack

It was a glorious day for golf—a sunny sky, clear with little humidity. Seventy-two-year-old Jack knew he was going to hit his best today. He met his buddies at the country club with a huge grin. "Today's my day," he said.

"Right, today's the day you shoot that hole-in-one!" they laughed. Jack had been threatening this for years. The

foursome had golfed together every Sunday afternoon for 15 years, swapping tales and good-natured ribbing.

But on this Sunday afternoon, when Jack bent down to insert his tee into the moist earth, he felt a sudden "crick" in his back. "Ow!" he said, grabbing his back. "I can't stand up straight."

"Man, that guy will do anything to get out of a bet," said one.

"Hang on," another said, seeing Jack stooped over in agony. "I don't think he's kidding."

Jack wasn't. And he received sobering news later that week from his doctor. Jack had broken a bone—the lower thoracic vertebra—in his spine, simply from bending over.

Since he retired five years earlier, one of Jack's greatest pleasures had been his days on the golf course, taking long walks down spacious greens chasing little white balls. Jack had quit a lifelong smoking habit and really felt his best years were ahead. That's what made the diagnosis of osteoporosis so frustrating. Just as Jack was fully embracing his retirement, he felt shortchanged and angry at his predicament.

"What? No way!" Jack practically barked at his doctor. "You have got to be kidding. Osteoporosis is a woman's disease—my wife has it!"

Coincidentally, Jack's wife Jenny had been devastated the year before to learn that she had suffered a spinal fracture from picking up one of her grandchildren. The proud grandmother of three had so looked forward to helping out with the energetic youngsters. But since her fracture, Jenny has been taking medication to decrease her risk of having another fracture and has been diligent about taking her calcium and vitamin D. She is determined to enjoy activities with her grandchildren in the years ahead. Jack was sobered to think that he could have osteoporosis too.

"Jack," the doctor said patiently, "osteoporosis doesn't only happen to women. It happens to men too. Unfortunately, many people don't understand the risks for osteoporosis in men. That's why those of us in the medical profession have such a difficult time educating people about the scope of this disease."

Jack is part of a growing number of men with osteoporosis. A 50-year-old white male like Jack has a 25 percent change of developing an osteoporosis-related fracture during his lifetime. By age 90, one in six men has suffered a hip fracture, often with devastating consequences.

Hormones and Bones

Both sexes rely on estrogens and androgens, the female and male "sex steroid" hormones, for bone health and strength. Testosterone plays an intricate role in calcium absorption, and, as the U.S. surgeon general reports, may stimulate bone formation even more than estrogen does. As men's androgen and estrogen levels start to taper off, they, too, become susceptible to age-related bone loss.

However, men start off with more bone tissue and maintain bone mass longer than women do. Plus, they don't experience the precipitous drop-off in bone density that women face at menopause, when female estrogen production grinds to a halt. Instead, the fall-off in male sex hormones occurs five to ten years down the road.

That may be why osteoporosis in men is *most often* associated with the following:

- Prolonged exposure to medications that impact bone density, including steroids, anticonvulsants, cancer therapies, aluminum-containing antacids
- Chronic illnesses that alter hormone levels, including kidney problems, lung conditions, ulcers, and other digestive problems
- Undiagnosed low levels of testosterone (hypogonadism)

That said, a family history of adult fractures is as important a risk factor for men as it is for women. And smoking, excessive drinking, low calcium intake, and a sedentary lifestyle negatively impact a man's bone health as much as a woman's.

The Bone Density Story for Men

Like all men, Jack's bone mineral density got a jump start during puberty, when his body began producing testosterone. Young men reach their peak spinal bone density by age 20. After that, they gradually lose about 30 percent of their trabecular bone, and 20 percent of their cortical bone, over the course of their lives.

Jack's actual bone loss most likely began during his 30s, when most men are oblivious to it. Scientists have documented a loss of bone minerals and bone density starting in the third decade of life. However, men generally maintain sufficient bone mass because the loss of bone largely keeps pace with bone rebuilding. This process continues, resulting in at least 1.5 million men over the age of 65 with osteoporosis.

Once men like Jack develop symptoms of osteoporosis, however, it's past time to see the doctor. Unfortunately, osteoporosis hits men particularly hard.

The risk of additional osteoporotic fractures increases after the first fracture for men as well as women. And as they age, both sexes face longer recuperation times and a loss of independence. But when men suffer a fracture, their health tends to spiral quickly downward into chronic disability. Hip and spinal fractures prove more deadly for men—older men are less likely than older women to survive a hip fracture, for example.

How Are Men's Risks of Osteoporosis Assessed?

Jack's doctor appropriately ordered a bone mineral density test for him after diagnosing a vertebral fracture. Medicare instituted coverage of bone density testing for the following groups of patients in 1998:

- Estrogen-deficient women at clinical risk for osteoporosis

- Individuals with vertebral abnormalities that on x-ray suggest osteoporosis, low bone mass, or vertebral fracture

- Individuals receiving long-term glucocorticoid (corticosteroid) therapy

- Individuals with primary hyperparathyroidism

- Individuals being monitored for their response to, or the effectiveness of, FDA-approved osteoporosis drug therapy

While Jack qualified for Medicare coverage, many men may question whether Medicare will cover their BMD tests. The guidelines above suggest that at-risk men do not yet enjoy the same preventive screening benefits as at-risk women. If you have questions about coverage, it is best to address them with your insurer.

Is It True That Vitamin D Deficiency Is Related to Osteoporosis in Men?

Vitamin D deficiency is being increasingly recognized as a common medical condition worldwide, but it has only recently been recognized as an epidemic. In April 2009, Eric Orwoll, MD, a widely published author in the area of male osteoporosis, released a study showing that 72 percent of men older than 65 throughout the United States had insufficient vitamin D levels. The study, published in the *Journal of Clinical Endocrinology & Metabolism* (94:1214–1222, 2009), noted that low vitamin D was most common in men living in northern sections of the country and that their levels were lowest during winter months. Those who reported outdoor activities had higher levels of vitamin D. Levels tended to be lower in the older men. This is not surprising, since aging decreases the skin's capacity to produce vitamin D and the presence of the precursor of vitamin D (7-dehydrocholesterol) also decreases with age.

In this study, obese men were more likely to have vitamin D deficiency. Vitamin D is a fat-soluble vitamin, and in normal-weight individuals, fat storage helps provide the vitamin D needed through the winter months when there is less sun exposure. However, both obese children and adults, defined as those with a body mass index over 30 kg/m^2 (kilograms per square meter), tend to sequester vitamin D in body fat. It may take twice the amount of vitamin D to maintain normal vitamin D levels in obese individuals than in those of normal weight.

The study noted that these multiple factors may be additive and stated that "in Caucasian men who were older than eighty years, with a BMI greater than 25 kg/m^2, who had vitamin D intake below 400 IU/d, did not engage in lawn/garden work, and who were sampled in winter or spring, the prevalence of vitamin D deficiency was 86 percent; whereas there was a prevalence of 24 percent in younger, thinner men who had higher vitamin D intakes, who were sampled in summer or fall, and who engaged in lawn/garden work." In summary, the vast majority of older sedentary men were found to have low vitamin D during winter months.

We can't keep from getting older, and most dermatologists advise sunscreen to decrease the risk of certain types of skin cancer, but we can be proactive about vitamin D intake and maintaining optimal body weight.

What Other Bone Loss "Triggers" Are There for Men?

When bone mineral density is lower than expected (even for men in their 70s like Jack) and the explanation eludes the doctor, further tests are often ordered.

Nearly 60 percent of men with osteoporosis have other disorders that produce bone loss, as we saw in chapter 3. Here are some examples of diseases that can trigger osteoporosis in men—on their own or over the course of their treatment.

Hypogonadism. Low testosterone production, or hypogonadism, affects bone strength in men as much as estrogen deficiency affects bone density in women. Hypogonadism can occur with few or no symptoms, making it particularly hard to detect in some men until osteoporosis sets in. Testosterone replacement therapy can correct this hormone deficiency.

Hyperparathyroidism. Hyperparathyroidism is the overactivity of the glands that secrete a hormone that maintains proper calcium levels in the blood and bones. Usually, the culprit is a growth on the parathyroid gland, which can be surgically removed.

Intestinal Disorders. Intestinal disorders that result in malabsorption can result in low bone density, osteoporosis, and fractures due to poor absorption of calcium, vitamin D, and other nutrients. Ulcerative colitis and Crohn's disease are inflammatory bowel diseases that are typically treated with corticosteroids to suppress painful inflammatory episodes. Adding calcium and vitamin D to the treatment regimen, as well as osteoporosis medications, is often recommended to offset bone loss from steroid use.

Prostate Cancer. This strictly male ailment is often treated with the GnRH agonist leuprolide to reduce androgen levels—predisposing men to low bone mass and fractures. Monitoring of bone density and appropriate treatment are recommended to prevent osteoporosis during treatment for prostate cancer.

Fighting a Male Myth

Many physicians fear that the misconception that men aren't at risk for osteoporosis may prevent many from seeking help early enough to benefit from preventive treatment. In most cases, calcium and vitamin D supplementation; weekly, monthly, or yearly osteoporosis medications; a safe weight-bearing exercise regimen; other lifestyle adjustments; and close follow-up with their physicians are successful in treating their osteoporosis or osteopenia, preventing bone loss, and protecting from future fractures.

That was just the prescription Jack received. His doctor prescribed medication, congratulated him on quitting smoking, and counseled him to limit his alcohol consumption and to take calcium supplements and vitamin D. The doctor also shared strategies for preventing falls.

Now Jack and Jenny are able to plan on a future in which they will continue their activities and enjoy an active lifestyle with their children and grandchildren.

Chapter 5

Assessing Bone Health

P revention may be the best strategy to combat the pending onslaught of osteoporosis that is predicted to hit like a wave as baby boomers age. However, unless you are fully convinced there's a real threat from osteoporosis, it's unlikely that you'll take steps to discover how healthy your bones really are, much less adopt preventive strategies.

Knowledge, as they say, is power. Today we have an arsenal of tests and information to help us diagnose and stave off this bone-thinning disease. Yet, even when we've got risk factors for osteoporosis, we tend to focus on other health issues, such as high cholesterol, overweight, and high blood pressure. These are all important, but it's unfortunate that most of us don't take our bone health as seriously.

Many people who are at risk for osteoporosis hesitate to schedule a BMD test—perhaps for fear that they may have to limit favorite activities or give up habits that may be unhealthy. Others may worry that their health insurance won't cover testing. It's more than worth your while to check with your insurer. And remember that Medicare covers BMD testing every two years for the indications we listed in chapter 3. Discussion is ongoing about expanding insurance coverage to include everyone at risk.

Frequently Asked Questions About Bone Health

Can Early Detection Really Make a Difference?

In the case of some diseases, there is little one can do to improve dramatically the situation once onset has occurred—but osteoporosis is not one of those diseases. Early detection offers so many advantages:

- You can begin taking medications that halt bone loss and build up bone mass, if needed.

- You can learn how to introduce more calcium into your diet and buttress your daily multivitamin with calcium and vitamin D supplements, all of which improve bone density.

- You can start a weight-bearing exercise program or tweak your workouts to include more weight-bearing activities, which strengthen bones.

- If you smoke, you'll have one more very good reason to quit.

How Will My Doctor Assess My Bone Health?

Physicians today are encouraged to look for signs of osteoporosis just as they do for heart disease, diabetes, and other problems during the yearly physical. This assessment of your overall health routinely includes checking height, weight, and spinal contour. A good doctor will assess many factors when evaluating your bone health, including the following.

Height

- Losing more than one and a half inches in height since age 21 may mean you have osteoporosis. Height loss can be the result of fractures of the vertebrae, the bones of the spine. Osteoporotic fractures of the spine may go undetected—about two-thirds of people with these fractures may not know that they have them, since their spine fractures were silent.

- Exceptional height is considered to be a risk

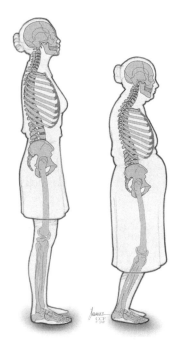

Vertebral compression fractures from osteoporosis can lead to kyphosis (curvature of the upper part of the spine) and height loss.

factor for osteoporosis by the American Society of Clinical Endocrinologists.

Weight

- If you weigh 127 pounds or less, your risk for osteoporosis is increased.

- Eating disorders, low body weight, and overexercise may result in osteoporosis.

Spinal Contour

- An increasing curvature of the spine with each passing year (kyphosis) points to loss of bone mass.

What Kind of Information Does My Doctor Need to Assess My Bone Health?

In addition to the factors listed previously, your physician will take a detailed personal and family medical history during your physical. Here are some questions your doctor may ask to determine your risks for osteoporosis:

Do you have an immediate relative who has suffered a fracture? The risk of hip fracture doubles for women whose mothers have had a hip fracture.

Do you have an immediate relative with osteoporosis or osteopenia? Bone fragility or fracture in a first-degree relative means that you may have inherited that same susceptibility.

Have you suffered recent fractures or falls? Three or more falls in one year raise your risks of fracture, particularly of the hip, and any woman who suffers a fracture after age 50 increases her risk of a hip fracture. Fractures, however, may be caused by other medical conditions, so a full evaluation by your doctor is critical.

Do you have an endocrine, kidney, or gastrointestinal disorder? Certain diseases and conditions are associated with loss of bone density.

Are you taking steroids or synthetic thyroid hormone? Taking prednisone in doses of 5 milligrams or more per day for more than three months to treat a medical condition can reduce your bone mass. Taking thyroid hormone for Graves's disease can raise risks of bone thinning if the dose is too high.

How much alcohol do you drink? Alcohol consumption of two or more drinks per day reduces bone density.

Do you smoke? Tobacco smoking—currently or in the past—is known to reduce bone mass, along with causing many other health problems.

Have you ever had an eating disorder? Anorexia nervosa or bulimia, especially during adolescence and young adulthood, can prevent you from achieving peak bone mass.

What is your menstrual history? Prolonged absence of periods due to excessive exercise, an eating disorder, or menopause can cause estrogen deficiency, which hastens loss of bone density. Premature menopause is an additional risk factor for osteoporosis. Late onset of menses may predispose a woman to low peak bone mass.

What is your diet like? Lifelong insufficient intake of calcium, vitamin D, or other nutrients can weaken your bones.

How much coffee do you drink? Excessive caffeine intake can rob the bones of key minerals.

What kind of exercise do you get? A sedentary lifestyle does nothing to strengthen bones; exercise must involve bearing weight to have a positive impact on bone health.

Have you ever had bariatric surgery? Gastric bypass and stomach stapling procedures can hamper absorption of calcium, vitamin D, and other nutrients our bones rely on.

Do you have chronic neck or back pain? Although there can be many causes of back and neck pain, these are sometimes symptoms of vertebral fracture.

If your answers to these questions suggest that you may be at increased risk for osteoporosis, then your doctor likely will recommend BMD testing.

Measuring Bone Density

Not so long ago, the only way to detect osteoporosis was when a bone fracture occurred or when you could literally see the disease progress, as the spine developed an increasing curvature. Today we have many tests at the ready; some measure bone mineral density, and others evaluate possible metabolic causes of bone loss.

Bone mineral density is one of the most important factors in predicting fracture risks from osteopenia and osteoporosis. BMD is routinely measured at the hip in women starting at age 65; men typically are screened starting at age 70.

Does Bone Density Testing Hurt?

Bone density testing is simple, it's painless, and it's the best way to determine your bone strength (weight-bearing capacity). Bone density can be measured at central sites, meaning the spine and hip, or at peripheral sites, such as the hand, heel, or wrist.

What Kind of Procedures Are Available for Bone Density Testing?

Currently, the major tests for measuring central bone mineral density include the following.

Dual-Energy X-Ray Absorptiometry (DXA). The World Health Organization considers DXA to be the gold standard in bone density testing. Indeed, DXA is the test that doctors most often recommend. Bone mineral density is calculated by dividing the amount of mineral content in a bone by the area or volume measured. Using two different low levels of x-ray energy, DXA can distinguish bone tissue from soft tissue in the spine, hip, or total body. DXA of the spine can provide earlier detection of osteoporosis than DXA of the hip and is recommended for younger postmenopausal women.

Quantitative Computed Tomography (QCT). This three-dimensional digital-imaging technique for measuring central bone density is used mainly in research studies. It measures true BMD volume in the hip or spine, analyzing trabecular (core) bone and cortical (outer) bone separately.

While QCT can very accurately detect early bone loss in spinal vertebrae, it isn't used as often as DXA because it is less able to predict actual fracture risk, is more costly, and exposes the patient to more radiation.

Quantitative Ultrasonography (QUS). QUS, or ultrasound densitometry, is the most recently arrived bone density measurement technique. Sound waves are transmitted through bone to spot reduced bone mineral content, usually at the kneecap or at the heel, which is composed of bone similar to that of the spine.

Ultrasound equipment is easily portable, costs little, and does not expose patients to any radiation. However, the American Medical Association recommends against its use in diagnosing osteopenia or osteoporosis or in monitoring patients' responses to treatment.

The main role of QUS—and it's an important one—is to serve as a mass screening tool to send lots of potentially at-risk individuals to the doctor for definitive diagnosis with DXA. For that reason, QUS is often used at community health fairs.

While central bone density testing is best at diagnosing osteoporosis and osteopenia—and the risk of spine and hip fractures—peripheral bone density tests can help to determine risks of fractures at other sites.

Peripheral DXA (pDXA). Peripheral DXA measures bone density and fracture risks in the wrist, heel, or finger.

Laboratory Tests. Tests that measure levels of vitamin D and other blood and urine tests may be ordered as important indicators of bone health. These are used in conjunction with DXA to determine your bone health, your risk of losing bone mass, and fracture risk.

In many centers, biochemical markers of bone turnover—which may be elevated in patients who are losing bone density and in those with osteoporosis—may become important predictors of fracture risks. However, these markers cannot yet be used accurately to diagnose osteoporosis.

Scoring Bone Mineral Density

The World Health Organization has used bone mineral density standards called T-scores and Z-scores to diagnose osteopenia and osteoporosis.

The T-score is also called the "young normal" score. It is calculated by comparing your bone mineral density to that of a healthy, same-sex 30-year-old (whose bone density is at its peak). The lower your T-score, the greater your risk of fracture.

The Z-score, also called the "age-matched" score, is used to compare your bone density to that of a healthy person of your age, gender, and build. Z-scores are not reliable in diagnosing osteoporosis because loss of bone density is common with age. However, high Z-scores frequently point to a

T-Scores

T-score: 1* or higher = normal bone mass.

T-score: −1 to −2.5 = osteopenia (low bone mass).

T-score: −2.5 or lower = osteoporosis.

T-score: −2.5 or lower with fracture = severe osteoporosis.

* A T-score of 1 means density within one standard deviation of the norm. Each standard deviation translates into a 10 to 12 percent loss in bone density. Osteopenia is diagnosed when scores fall between 1 and 2.5 standard deviations below normal. Osteoporosis is diagnosed when scores drop 2.5 standard deviations below the norm.

secondary cause of osteoporosis, such as steroid use, hyperparathyroidism, or vitamin D deficiency.

What's All This About FRAX?

Until recently, most clinical guidelines that physicians used to make recommendations about the management of osteoporosis were based on the T-score. While treatment was always recommended for people who had a fragility fracture (a fracture that occurs with a fall from standing height or lower), the decision about which patients should be prescribed medications was based on the T score as derived from the DXA bone density test.

However, experts noted that other factors in the patient's history were powerful predictors of future fractures and needed to be taken into account in treatment guidelines. For instance, age is an important factor that predicts the likelihood of fracture. The hip fracture risk quadruples between the ages of 55 and 85, so T-score alone may not be the best way to make treatment decisions. As a result of an important international initiative, the WHO Collaborating Centre for Metabolic Bone Diseases has developed international guidelines that predict an individual's risk of fracture over the next ten years. This algorithm, referred to as FRAX, was released in 2008. It incorporates many clinical conditions, is computer and Web based, and can be individualized by country and racial group. It can then be used to advise physicians all over the world about whom would be most appropriate to treat with osteoporosis medications.

The clinical conditions that are taken into account in the new FRAX guidelines include the following:

- Prior fragility fracture
- Parental history of hip fracture
- Current tobacco smoking
- Long-term use of oral glucocorticoids
- Rheumatoid arthritis
- Other causes of secondary osteoporosis
- Daily alcohol consumption of three or more units

At present, FRAX models are available for Austria, China, Germany, France, Italy, Japan, Spain, Sweden, Switzerland, Turkey, the United Kingdom, and the United States. In the United States, the National Osteoporosis Foundation has incorporated the FRAX into its official treatment guidelines.

Using FRAX

You can access the FRAX WHO Fracture Risk Assessment Tool by going to *www.shef.ac.uk/FRAX/*. You can plug in your age, sex, height, weight, answers to the questions relating to your clinical history, and your bone density, and you can then see the calculation for your ten-year percentage probability of a major osteoporotic fracture and a hip fracture specifically. This model applies to men and women over the age of 50 who have never been on osteoporosis medication. This model is continually being updated as new data are incorporated into the algorithm.

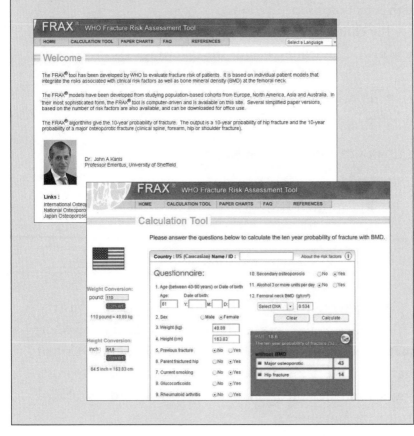

National Osteoporosis Foundation Treatment Guidelines

The 2008 National Osteoporosis Foundation treatment guidelines recommend initiation of pharmacologic therapy to reduce fracture risk in postmenopausal women and men 50 years of age or older with the following risk factors:

- A hip or vertebral (clinical or morphometric) fracture

- A T score of less than or equal to −2.5 by central DXA at the femoral neck, total hip, or spine

- Low bone mass and a ten-year probability of fracture of 3 percent or more, or a ten-year probability of any major osteoporosis-related fracture of 20 percent or over, based on the U.S.-adapted WHO FRAX algorithm.

Your Bone Health Is Your Responsibility

Ask your physician about your fracture risk and need for treatment.

Chapter 6

Managing Osteoporosis

Not so long ago, people like Kate and Jack had every reason to fear a diagnosis of osteoporosis. In the 1950s, little could be done to treat the disease, let alone prevent it or halt its progression.

But times have changed.

No longer does a diagnosis of osteoporosis signal that it's time to pack up your belongings and move to a nursing home for fear of falls and fractures when you're alone.

It's a different world today—people are living longer than ever. Many of us expect to encounter health problems along the way. A diagnosis such as osteoporosis doesn't have the same impact, because progress in medicine has given us reason to hope—and concrete means of coping.

With an accurate diagnosis and a thorough prevention or treatment plan, people with osteopenia and osteoporosis are leading healthy, productive lives. They are eating well, exercising, and increasing their calcium intake. Many are taking prescription medicine to improve their bone density. Doctors are tracking their progress with noninvasive, quick, painless tests.

Because of growing interest in the area of osteoporosis, exciting studies about new treatment options are published almost monthly.

Let's put these new treatments into context by looking at the various forms of osteoporosis treatment used over the years.

Early Treatment with Estrogen

Thirty years ago, estrogen therapy (ET) was routinely prescribed to boost waning hormone levels among menopausal women—both to prevent osteoporosis and to control menopausal symptoms such as hot flashes, night sweats, sleep deprivation, and mood swings. When heart disease emerged as a leading killer among postmenopausal women, doctors believed that estrogen therapy would protect the heart as well.

As time went on, physicians discovered that ET alone had other, less welcome, effects. It increased the risk of cancer of the uterine lining (the endometrium), except, of course, in women who had undergone hysterectomy.

To protect women with an intact uterus from endometrial cancer, progestin was added to estrogen. The female hormone combination was dubbed HRT, for hormone replacement therapy. HRT renews a menopausal woman's menstrual cycle.

Isn't Hormone Replacement Therapy Dangerous?

In 2002, the National Institutes of Health released the results of the Women's Health Initiative (WHI) study. Tracking 15,000 women between the ages of 50 and 79, the study found that women on HRT had a higher incidence of breast cancer, heart disease, and stroke. HRT was quickly suspended among women in the study. The storm of publicity that followed caused panic among many women taking HRT for menopausal symptoms. They abandoned the therapy in droves, and many doctors stopped prescribing it. As a result, the decision by many women to forgo HRT may have contributed to the growing incidence of osteoporosis.

The progestin component of HRT may have been the culprit in the risk of heart attack and stroke. The WHI later confirmed that ET alone caused no ill effects among women

HRT: What You Didn't Hear

Initial media reports on the WHI hormone replacement therapy findings downplayed three key factors:

1. Only one HRT preparation (PREMPRO) was studied among the many forms and dosages available.

2. Many study participants began HRT in their 60s, long past the time women typically need relief from menopausal symptoms.

3. Women in the study were on HRT for five years, so the effects of shorter-term therapy were not considered.

who had undergone hysterectomy. Low-dose ET is approved for the prevention of bone loss in postmenopausal women, and may be a reasonable option for those not at risk of endometrial cancer due to hysterectomy.

The Bottom Line. The U.S. Food and Drug Administration (FDA) no longer recommends HRT or ET as a *primary* treatment for bone loss. Instead, the FDA advises women who choose to take HRT or ET for menopausal symptoms to *take the lowest possible dose for the least amount of time required.*

It is critical for every woman considering HRT to meet with her physician to review carefully all of her individual risk factors. If osteoporosis is her main concern, therapies are now available that zero in on bone loss without carrying the baggage of HRT.

Current Medication Options

So what's available today to strengthen thinning bones? Options are rapidly expanding on the medication front. Any medication should be given along with a regimen of appropriate calcium and vitamin D. The two types of medications that are presently available for treatment of osteopenia and osteoporosis are *antiresorptives* and *anabolic* medications.

Bisphosphonates, calcitonin, estrogen, and selective estrogen receptor modulators (SERMs) are medications that specifically inhibit the bone-dissolving activity of osteoclasts. These are classified as antiresorptive medications.

Another medication, which is a form of parathyroid hormone (PTH), represents a totally different class of medication—the first bone-building anabolic agent to be approved by the FDA

Each osteoporosis medication has its strengths and its drawbacks, so it is important that your physician select the one that is right for you.

When Are Bisphosphonates Prescribed to Treat Osteoporosis?

Bisphosphonates are considered the first line of defense in treating a variety of bone disorders. These medications cannot be used in people with renal (kidney) insufficiency or with certain other medical conditions involving abnormal calcium metabolism. They cannot be used during pregnancy. They are approved by the FDA for women after menopause as well as in men over the age of 50 who have osteoporosis. This class of drugs includes alendronate, risedronate, ibandronate, and zoledronic acid and can be given on a daily, weekly, monthly, or yearly basis.

- **Alendronate** (Fosamax). This drug targets long-term bone loss. The International Osteoporosis Foundation (IOF) reports that this well-studied drug, available since 1995, increases overall bone mineral density and reduces hip and spine fractures by about 50 percent. Alendronate is prescribed for postmenopausal women at risk of osteoporosis and for men with low bone density. It is also prescribed for people with osteoporosis resulting from steroid (prednisone or cortisone) therapy. Alendronate is available in daily and weekly dosages and is now available in a generic form.

- **Risedronate** (Actonel). This drug became available in 2000 and is used both for the prevention and the treatment of osteoporosis. The IOF reports that risedronate increases bone mineral density while slowing bone loss in postmenopausal women and reduces risks of spine and hip fractures by 40 to 50 percent. It is used to prevent bone loss and fractures in patients on steroids. Prescribed for men as well as women, risedronate can also treat osteoporosis stemming from long-term use of medications that cause osteoporosis. It is available in daily and weekly dosages.

- **Ibandronate** (Boniva). This drug, approved in early 2005 for the treatment of osteoporosis, specifically targets the spine. Studies show that ibandronate increases bone mineral density in the spine and reduces vertebral fracture risk. Monthly oral doses of ibandronate are available. This medication can also be administered intravenously in a doctor's office every three months.

- **Zoledronic acid** (Reclast). This drug is a yearly intravenous bisphosphonate that has been shown to reduce the risk of hip, vertebral, and nonvertebral fractures. It has also been shown to decrease subsequent fractures in patients who have already had an osteoporosis-related fracture and to increase the survival of those who have sustained a low-trauma hip fracture. Zoledronic acid has been shown to be effective for the prevention and treatment of bone loss that is associated with glucocorticoid use.

Check with your doctor and pharmacist for further details and help in selecting the best formulation for you. Like any other medication, bisphosphonates have side effects. These are infrequent but include muscle and joint aches, stomach upset, and heartburn.

To ensure proper absorption, oral bisphosphonates should be taken with water on an empty stomach first thing in the morning. It's important not to lie down for 30 to 60 minutes after taking oral bisphosphonates to decrease risks of esophageal irritation.

Are Bisphosphonates Safe? The answer, for the vast majority of people with osteoporosis, is that the benefits of bisphosphonates far outweigh their risks. You may have heard or read stories in the media about bone medications causing osteonecrosis of the jaw (ONJ). ONJ involves the death of bone tissue in the jaw, causing jaw pain and even exposing bone. But osteonecrosis of the jaw is a *rare* condition—it is less likely to occur in patients on osteoporosis treatment with bisphosphonates than getting struck by lightning! In rare circumstances, it affects individuals on high-dose intravenous bisphosphonates for cancer (typically, myeloma, breast cancer, or prostate cancer).

Among the several million people taking lower-dose oral bisphosphonates for osteoporosis, only a few hundred cases have been reported worldwide, usually after invasive dental procedures like extractions.

Nevertheless, precautions are wise. In June 2006, the American Dental Association recommended a comprehensive oral evaluation before—or as soon as possible after—starting oral bisphosphonate therapy. Good oral hygiene and regular dental care are critical. The American College of Rheumatology further recommends that before taking bisphosphonates, patients should complete any traumatic dental treatments, such as tooth extractions. Any jaw pain or dental pain should be evaluated periodically during bisphosphonate treatment.

What Treatments Are Currently Available Besides Bisphosphonate Therapy?

The following list includes descriptions of some alternatives to bisphosphonate therapy.

Calcitonin (Miacalcin). Calcitonin has been available as a treatment for osteoporosis of the spine since 1986. Calcitonin is a hormone secreted by the thyroid gland that regulates calcium metabolism along with parathyroid hormone. Studies show that administering calcitonin may slow bone loss in the spine, increase spinal bone density by 1 to 2 percent, and reduce spinal fractures. Some women with osteoporosis report that calcitonin reduces spine pain.

Unfortunately, calcitonin apparently does nothing to reduce fractures in the hip or elsewhere. Initially available only in injectable form, calcitonin was introduced in a nasal spray form in 1995. It is taken once a day, at any time. Side effects include a runny or stuffy nose, and allergic reactions have occurred with the injectable form.

SERMs (Raloxifene/Evista). Selective estrogen receptor modulators, or SERMs, are estrogen analogs, produced in the laboratory to mimic estrogen's beneficial effect on bone while blocking its deleterious effects on breast and uterine tissue.

Raloxifene (Evista), introduced in 1999, is the only SERM available for preventing and treating vertebral fractures in postmenopausal women. Studies show that three years of raloxifene treatment will reduce the risks of spine fractures by 30 to 50 percent and will increase bone density in the spine and hip by 2 to 3 percent. Because raloxifene does not protect against fractures elsewhere in the body, it is not considered potent enough to reduce the risk of hip and other nonvertebral fractures. Raloxifen is taken by mouth once a day, at any time.

Side effects of this estrogen analog include intensified hot flashes, increased leg cramps, and a small risk of clot formation. Thus, raloxifene is not a good option for anyone who is at increased risk of stroke, pulmonary embolism, or deep vein thrombosis. It is also not recommended if patients will be immobilized for a prolonged period of time—due to surgery and recovery, for example, or lengthy travel.

Raloxifene has been shown to decrease the risk of invasive breast cancer in some patients at high risk for breast cancer, so it may be an option for some patients with a positive family history of breast cancer who also have spinal osteopenia but who are not at high risk for hip or other nonvertebral fractures.

Other SERMs with slightly different chemical actions are also under study.

Parathyroid Hormone Derivatives (Teriparatide/Forteo). Parathyroid hormone (PTH) has unique bone-forming capabilities that scientists have known about for more than

70 years. PTH is secreted by the parathyroid gland and plays a key role in calcium and bone metabolism. An active form of the hormone was not introduced as a medication until 2002. A multinational study has found that synthetic PTH reduces vertebral fractures by 65 percent and nonspinal fractures by 53 percent among postmenopausal women.

Teriparatide (Forteo) is the only FDA-approved medication derived from PTH to become available to date, although other formulations are anticipated. Teriparatide increases bone density while stimulating new bone growth. Studies show that teriparatide, approved for males and females at high risk of fractures, reduces spine, hip, foot, rib, and wrist fractures in postmenopausal women and spine fractures in men.

Teriparatide may be given by daily injection for no longer than two years, due to FDA concerns about bone cancer in rats exposed to large doses over long periods of time. It should be avoided by patients with other bone diseases, such as Paget's disease; those with unexplained increases in alkaline phosphate or blood calcium levels; patients who are young and actively forming new bone; and anyone with a history of bone cancer or radiation therapy to the bone.

Emerging Medications

Scientists continue to research new osteoporosis drugs that act in entirely different capacities than current formulations. They are also investigating novel ways of delivering standard medications. We will discuss some emerging medical therapies in chapter 9.

Surgical Options

Why would anyone require surgery for osteoporosis? Because minimally invasive surgery can relieve the pain of compression fractures in the small bones of the spine.

Someone fractures a vertebra approximately every 45 seconds in the United States. Vertebral compression fractures account for nearly half of the 1.5 million "fragility fractures" that occur annually. Osteoporosis is almost always the culprit. While most vertebral fractures affect postmenopausal women, men are not immune.

When vertebrae are fragile, they can fracture from activities as harmless as rolling over in bed or getting out of a car. The vertebrae are normally stacked one on top of the other in the spinal column, separated by discs. When vertebrae collapse or fracture, their height may be compressed by 15 to 20 percent or more. This results in pain, as vertebrae press against their neighbors; in loss of height; and in problems with walking and balance.

After successive vertebral fractures heal, they create a forward spinal curvature called kyphosis (in the past, a "dowager's hump"). In severe kyphosis, the chest cavity shrinks, limiting the lungs' capacity to expand. Pneumonia and other respiratory problems may ensue.

Are There Procedures to Repair an Injured Spine?

Several procedures are available for repairing an injured spine:

Vertebroplasty involves inserting a needle into a recently fractured veretebra. Bone cement is then injected to seal the break.

Kyphoplasty involves inserting a needle into the space between collapsed vertebrae and introducing a balloonlike device, which is then inflated. The balloon is withdrawn, and the newly expanded space is filled with bone cement.

Both vertebroplasty and kyphoplasty can potentially stabilize and straighten the spine, with many positive effects. In some studies, patients reported improved physical function, increased vitality and socialization, an improved outlook, and a reduction in pain after minimally invasive treatment for kyphosis. Long-term studies on the safety and efficacy of these procedures are ongoing. However, two recent released studies showed no differences in pain or disability in patients who were treated with vertebroplasty when compared to patients getting a "sham" procedure. Additional studies are ongoing.

It's In Your Hands

There are many treatment options that can strengthen bones and decrease the risk of subsequent fractures, even in patients with severe osteoporosis. I have had many patients plagued by one fracture after another who are now able to live active and independent lives, thanks to these bone-building and fracture-preventing medications.

But in addition to treatment your doctor may provide, there will always be elements you must take responsibility for. Part of any good treatment plan includes strengthening your bones from the inside out, so we'll learn how to do that in the next chapter.

Chapter 7

Protecting Yourself from the Inside Out

You can improve your bone health through simple but significant changes in diet, exercise habits, and life-style. A well-rounded diet helps to ensure a good supply of the nutrients and vitamins we need for healthy bones.

Calcium and vitamin D, which helps our bodies absorb calcium, are considered the cornerstones of bone health. The more calcium we take in during childhood, the greater our bone mass will be when we reach adulthood. And the higher our bone mass, the lower the risk for fractures. So it's important to start paying attention to calcium intake early. But even if you didn't get enough calcium in childhood, it's not too late—our bone tissue continues to replace itself every ten years, so in reality our bodies need a constant supply of calcium, not just a big influx at the beginning.

A Starting Point

A report in *The New England Journal of Medicine* in February, 16, 2006, may have created some confusion by suggesting that calcium and vitamin D are less helpful to postmenopausal women than previously believed. In a group of healthy post-menopausal women, researchers found that calcium and vitamin D supplementation slightly improved hip bone density but did *not* significantly reduce the number of hip fractures.

That is when medications, such as the bisphosphonates described in the previous chapter, are so useful. Joel S. Finkelstein, MD, spelled it out best in his accompanying editorial: "Calcium with vitamin D supplementation is akin to the ante for a poker game: it is where everyone starts. If the clinical data suggest that the risk of fracture is significant, however, a woman probably needs something more."

Your best option is to take the daily recommended amounts of calcium and vitamin D while realizing that they cannot prevent fractures on their own. If you have any concerns, talk them over with your doctor.

How Much Calcium Do We Really Need?

Calcium not only helps maintain healthy bones. It also helps keep our hearts pumping, our nerves firing, and our blood clotting properly. So there's no question that we need adequate amounts. But actual calcium requirements vary by age. The

National Osteoporosis Foundation recommends following these guidelines from The National Academy of Sciences:

Recommended Daily Calcium Intake

Infants
Birth to six months: 210 milligrams
Six months to one year: 270 milligrams

Children/Young Adults
One to three years: 500 milligrams
Four to eight years: 800 milligrams
Nine to eighteen years: 1,300 milligrams

Adult Women and Men
Nineteen to fifty years: 1,000 milligrams
Fifty-plus years: 1,200 milligrams

Pregnant or Lactating Women
Eighteen years or younger: 1,300 milligrams
Nineteen to fifty years: 1,000 milligrams

The recommended calcium intake for postmenopausal women who are not taking estrogen is 1,500 milligrams daily, according to some experts. Individuals with a history of calcium kidney stones should consult with their physicians about appropriate calcium intake and supplementation.

Can I Take in More Calcium Just by Changing My Diet?

Luckily for us, calcium is found in many foods. Calcium-rich foods include dairy products such as milk, yogurt, cheese, and even ice cream; shellfish; vegetables such as spinach and broccoli; nuts; and soy products, including tofu. You'll find a comprehensive list of foods high in calcium at the end of this chapter.

• • • *Fast Fact* • • •

The amount of calcium that we absorb varies by food source. More calcium is absorbed from dairy products than from vegetables, for instance.

• • •

The Importance of Balance

Getting the right amount of nutrients in our diet can sometimes be tricky because some foods impede our ability to get the most out of others. For example, to help with calcium metabolism, we need to get the right amount of protein into our systems. Studies link low protein intake to problems with calcium absorption and high protein intake to increased urinary excretion of calcium. Two to three servings of protein a day, in the form of meat, poultry, beans, or dairy, are all we need.

Dietary sodium (salt) has also come under the scrutiny of osteoporosis researchers. Higher-sodium diets

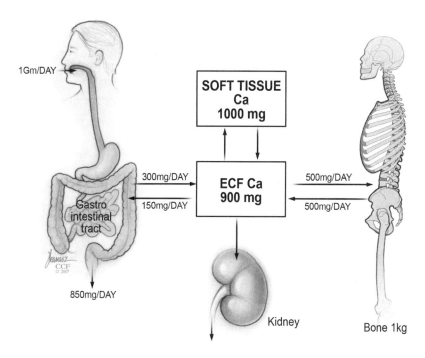

Calcium metabolism involves an exquisite balance between dietary intake, intestinal absorption, and excretion by the kidneys all interacting through the blood calcium level with the bones of the skeleton.

increase calcium output in the urine—and bone resorption as a result. However, replacing the lost calcium through supplementation appears to offset bone loss.

As we discussed in chapter 1, it's also important to go easy on the soft drinks, especially for younger people. The phosphorus and caffeine that many contain—and not just the colas—can throw off your calcium balance and negatively impact your bone health. Furthermore, high phosphate intake increases parathyroid hormone (PTH) secretion. As we've read, PTH is one of the hormones that regulates calcium levels in our bones. And excess PTH is the culprit in hyperparathyroidism, which causes excessive bone resorption and secondary osteoporosis.

But even a well-rounded diet of vegetables, proteins, fruits, and grains may not provide all the calcium that we need. And the truth is, many of us do not always eat well-balanced meals with our hectic schedules and eating on the run.

Choosing the Right Calcium Supplement

If your doctor tells you to take calcium, unless you are able to incorporate the entire recommended amount into your dietary intake on a daily basis, it's time to head to the pharmacy. No problem—calcium supplements are relatively inexpensive and easy to find, right?

Suddenly you're standing in a drugstore with rows of calcium supplements staring you in the face. With so many forms and dosages available, is one better than the other?

So How Do I Choose a Calcium Supplement?

First of all, look for calcium supplements labeled "purified" or displaying the United States Pharmacopoeia (USP) symbol. Then consider the source: calcium is derived from several.

Calcium Citrate. Calcium citrate (in Citracal and other brands) is often recommended as the best and most readily absorbed form of calcium supplementation. *Citrate* means that the calcium is derived from citric acid (found in citrus fruit). Calcium is best absorbed in an acidic environment in the stomach, such as around meal time, but calcium citrate provides an acidic formulation, so it is well-absorbed at anytime. Since it is well-absorbed even when not taken with food, it is more convenient, although it is frequently more expensive than some other calcium supplements.

Calcium Carbonate. Calcium carbonate is another common form of calcium. It is refined from limestone, oyster shell, or other shell sources and must be taken with food. Because of its antacid properties, calcium carbonate is also used in products like Tums. It's important to note that calcium carbonate also reduces the amount of iron absorbed from food by as much as 50 percent.

Other Sources. Less common sources of calcium include calcium gluconate, calcium lactate, and calcium phosphate—all less well absorbed than calcium citrate.

How Many Calcium Supplement Pills Should I Be Taking?

Daily intake recommendations on the bottle refer to the amount of *elemental* calcium the product contains. This differs, depending on the source.

For example, calcium citrate is 21 percent elemental calcium. That means you'll get 210 milligrams of elemental calcium from 1,000 milligrams of calcium citrate. Calcium carbonate is 40 percent elemental calcium, however, so you'll get 400 milligrams of elemental calcium from 1,000 milligrams of calcium carbonate.

So you may need different numbers of pills to meet your daily calcium requirement. If you aren't comfortable swallowing a lot of pills every day, choose extra-strength supplements or chewable or liquid forms.

Whichever calcium supplement you choose, it's best to divide your overall daily dose so that you're taking about 500 milligrams at a time to maximize absorption. But if you wind up taking your entire daily dose at once, that's still better than taking no calcium at all.

Do Calcium Supplements Have Any Side Effects?

Calcium supplements can cause gastrointestinal problems, including constipation. Switching between preparations may eliminate those problems. If you find it difficult to tolerate *any* calcium supplements, speak to your doctor about alternatives.

Don't Forget the Vitamin D

Natural sunlight is our main source of vitamin D. Yet our ability to absorb this vitamin varies according to climate, how much sunscreen and clothing we wear, our pigmentation (darker-skinned individuals take longer to convert sunlight into vitamin D), and our age (the older we are, the less efficiently our skin makes active vitamin D). According to the National Osteoporosis Foundation, adults who are 50 and older need 800–1000 IU of vitamin D per day, and adults under 50 need 400–800 IU. However, recommendations vary.

The Recommended Daily Allowance (RDA) developed by the Institute of Medicine of the national Academy of Sciences recommends an Adequate Intake (AI) of vitamin D of 400 IU daily for adults 51–70 and 600 IU for those over age 71. The recommended RDA for birth to age 50 is 200 IU. However, many sources recommend much higher levels of intake for optimal bone health as well as to support multiple other body functions, including immune function, muscle strength and even possible cancer prevention. An article by Reinhold Vieth in the *American Journal of Clinical Nutrition* (69:842–859, 1999) recommended 4,000 IU of vitamin D per day for adults and cited data that vitamin D toxicity is rare. Vitamin D2 is less potent than the natural active form, vitamin D3.

While some foods, particularly fatty fish (salmon, sardines, mackerel), vitamin D–fortified milk, and other foods fortified with vitamin D, can help us increase the vitamin D in our diets, most people will need to take a vitamin D supplement to get to the National Osteoporosis Foundation (NOF) recommendation of 1,000 IU of vitamin D per day. Some countries have routinely supplemented products like margarine in an attempt to increase the average vitamin D levels in their citizens. More studies are needed on vitamin D intake and the role it plays in many body functions.

Many studies show that most American women do *not* get adequate vitamin D, and multiple professional organizations have emphasized the important role that physicians should play in counseling patients about vitamin D intake.

Insufficient levels of vitamin D increase bone turnover and susceptibility to fractures. Vitamin D deficiency is linked not just to osteoporosis but also to a variety of other bone disorders, including rickets.

Vitamin D Recommendations

How, Exactly, Does Vitamin D Improve My Bone Health?

Vitamin D boosts our bone health in several ways:

- Aiding the absorption of calcium from the gastro-intestinal tract
- Controlling calcium excretion by the kidneys
- Directly affecting cells in the bone by interacting with receptors on osteoblasts

An International Osteoporosis Foundation report has suggested that calcitrol, the active portion of vitamin D, may help stimulate bone-forming osteoblasts and reduce the likelihood of spine fractures after menopause. In another study, vitamin D plus calcium significantly increased hip bone density and decreased the fracture rate among elderly women. Yet nearly 50 percent of women over age 70 do not meet their daily requirements for vitamin D.

How Much Vitamin D Should I Be Getting Each Day?

The National Osteoporosis Foundation recommends that adults under age 50 need 400–800 IU of vitamin D daily and adults who are 50 and older need 800–1,000 IU of vitamin D daily. Vitamin D may be taken on its own or combined with calcium. However, if your physician finds in your blood tests that your vitamin D level is very low, you may be prescribed much higher doses, so check with your doctor about your vitamin D needs.

Next Step: Get Moving!

Exercise is a key component of physical and mental well-being at all ages. The U.S. surgeon general calls for a lifelong commitment to maintaining bone health through exercise. Stopping an exercise program completely will cause us to lose any gains we've realized in bone mass. So variety and creativity are important to maintain our interest.

Research shows that the greatest long-term gains in bone mass happen when we exercise during our youth. However, we face tall hurdles in moving beyond our social and cultural lethargy:

- Schools are cutting exercise and gym classes from curricula.
- Television, playing video games, and chatting on the Internet cheat youngsters of the time they might spend on physical activity instead.

Thus, it's more important than ever for parents and caregivers to keep children on the move. Of course, balance is important: there is such a thing as too much exercise. Adolescent girls who exercise to the point where they see a precipitous drop in body weight and a cessation of periods deprive their growing bones of needed estrogen.

Research is unclear about how much exercise provides the best long-term benefit for bone health at different ages. Exercise alone, or with calcium supplementation, may not be able to prevent bone density from plummeting during menopause.

But what is clear is that regular, weight-bearing exercise builds bone mass, strengthens muscles, and stabilizes the skeleton, improving balance and coordination. Weight-bearing exercise provides a greater-than-normal stimulus to bones by making them work against gravity.

With a sturdy musculoskeletal system, we are much more likely to ward off devastating fractures and costly falls as we age.

What Kind of Exercise Should I Be Doing to Promote Bone Health, and How Much?

We recommend the following exercise guidelines, adapted from the U.S. surgeon general's *Report on Bone Health and Osteoporosis*.

For children over eight and adolescents: A healthy exercise program includes 60 minutes of moderately intense activity every day. Weight-bearing activities that gradually increase bone strength include running, hopping, or skipping, along with intense sports that involve short bursts of jumping, like basketball, gymnastics, soccer, and volleyball. Swimming and bicycling, while excellent forms of exercise, are not weight-bearing activities and do not build bone mass.

For adults: A good exercise program includes at least 30 minutes of physical activity a day. (Cleaning your house, gardening, or raking are not substitutes for daily exercise.) Strength training combined with short, intermittent periods

of aerobic activity seems to work best for improving bone health. So incorporate strength or resistance training into workouts at least twice a week. Activities to consider include walking, jogging, climbing stairs, hiking, weight training, aerobics, dancing, and sports such as basketball and tennis that require lots of running and jumping. For patients with limitations on their activity dictated by arthritis or cardiac or pulmonary diseases, working closely with a physican and a physical therapist can help them find their optimal activity and exercise routine.

For older adults: It's important to maintain as much muscle mass as possible since poor muscle strength is a known risk factor for falls. Physical activity of 30 to 45 minutes, three times a week for at least three months, has been shown to improve both strength and balance. Even limited strength and resistance exercises can build muscle mass. Weight-bearing movement activities, such as tai chi, can enhance balance and coordination and stimulate bone. Many senior centers and hospitals offer wonderful exercise programs tailored to elderly individuals' needs. Again, consultation with your physican and referral to a physical therapist may be the best way to keep you active and improve your bone health.

Do I Need to Involve My Doctor in My Exercise Program?

With any exercise program, it's best to ask your doctor about any restrictions or recommendations before you start, especially if you have already been diagnosed with a bone disease or another illness. Your physician may recommend that you see a physical therapist to help you develop an exercise

Too Busy to Exercise?

Women pressed with competing demands at home and at work often struggle to find the time and make a commitment to an exercise routine. Exercising will not only protect women's bones, it will also boost energy and improve mood.

The American College of Sports Medicine states that, for women,

- weight-bearing physical activity is essential to developing and maintaining a healthy skeleton;

- weight-bearing exercise can increase bone mass slightly in sedentary women but, more importantly, can prevent further bone loss from inactivity; and

- the ideal exercise program incorporates activities that increase strength, flexibility, and coordination to decrease risks of falls and fractures.

program that's safe and effective for you. Physical therapists will tailor exercises to your individual needs. For elderly individuals, they will make sure that exercises don't impact balance, a key consideration.

Lifestyle Considerations

Finally, to maximize bone health, we really need to look at the entire spectrum of our lifestyle behaviors—including smoking and drinking.

Drinking alcohol inhibits bone formation. While some studies show that moderate alcohol consumption increases bone density, there is as yet no evidence that drinking reduces fracture risks. Indeed, higher alcohol consumption increases the likelihood of falls and ensuing fractures.

Smoking also has direct and indirect effects on bone. The chemicals in cigarettes, including nicotine, are toxic to bone, lowering calcium absorption from the gastrointestinal tract and altering levels of vitamin D. Smoking also decreases body weight and absorbs hormones needed for bone strength, further increasing our susceptibility to fractures.

When we smoke and drink to excess, we tend to be less physically active, compounding our risk of fractures. Fortunately, it is never too late to stop smoking and to modify our alcohol intake.

Teaming Up with Your Doctor

As doctors, we can examine you physically and assess your health using various tests. But no one knows your body better than you. If you have any health concerns, we want to hear them. It's much better to ask questions than to guess.

Make a list of your questions and concerns between visits to the doctor. Do you notice any altered function? Do you have pain where you didn't before? Are you confused about when to take your calcium and vitamin D, or are the side effects bothersome?

Together, we are a team. We can take steps to improve your bone health, track your progress and—as we'll see in the next chapter—adopt smart strategies for prevention.

Selected Calcium-Rich Foods

FOOD	CALCIUM (MG)
Fortified oatmeal, 1 packet	350
Sardines, canned in oil, with edible bones, 3 oz.	324
Cheddar cheese, 1½ oz. shredded	306
Milk, nonfat, 1 cup	302
Milkshake, 1 cup	300
Yogurt, plain, low-fat, 1 cup	300
Soybeans, cooked, 1 cup	261
Tofu, firm, with calcium, ½ cup	204*
Orange juice, fortified with calcium, 6 oz.	200–260 (varies)
Salmon, canned, with edible bones, 3 oz.	181
Pudding, instant (chocolate, banana, etc.) made with 2% milk, ½ cup	153
Baked beans, 1 cup	142
Cottage cheese, 1% milk fat, 1 cup	138
Spaghetti, lasagna, 1 cup	125
Frozen yogurt, vanilla, soft-serve, ½ cup	103
Ready-to-eat cereal, fortified with calcium, 1 cup	100–1,000 (varies)
Cheese pizza, 1 slice	100
Fortified waffles, 2	100
Turnip greens, boiled, ½ cup	99
Broccoli, raw, 1 cup	90
Ice cream, vanilla, ½ cup	85
Soy or rice milk, fortified with calcium, 1 cup	80–500 (varies)

Source: *The 2004 Surgeon General's Report on Bone Health and Osteoporosis: What It Means to You*. U.S. Department of Health and Human Services, Office of the Surgeon General, 2004, pages 12–13.

* The calcium content of tofu may vary depending on processing methods. Tofu processed with calcium salts can have as much as 300 milligrams for every 4 ounces. Often, the label or the manufacturer can provide more specific information.

Note: You may also increase the calcium in foods by these suggestions:

- Add nonfat powdered milk to all soups, casseroles, and drinks.
- Buy juices, cereals, and breads that are fortified with calcium.
- Replace whole milk and cream with skim and low-fat milk in recipes.
- Replace sour cream with yogurt in recipes.
- Some bottled waters contain calcium, so check the labels for more information.

Source: USDA Nutrient Data Laboratory

Chapter 8

Preventing Falls and Fractures

H ere's an all too common story.

On a short flight from Cleveland to New York City, Helen just finishes rehearsing her PowerPoint presentation on her laptop computer as the plane taxis to a stop. Ever the efficient professional, she's packed everything she needs (and more) in her carry-on, now stowed in the overhead compartment. Though the bag meets the airline's weight limits, Helen is not a big woman. In fact, she's slender and willowy. When the seatbelt sign goes off, she goes to take her bag down from the overhead bin. Suddenly, she feels a sharp zing in the middle of her back.

What's that? she wonders, dragging the bag down and reaching around with her hand to her bra line. Assuming she's just pulled a muscle, Helen edges into the aisle, gingerly pulling her tote behind her as she and the other passengers disembark the plane.

Putting the incident behind her, Helen continues to note significant pain, which gradually improves over the next several weeks. However, she carries on and dives quickly back into her hectic work schedule. She doesn't even see her doctor until later that year, when a cold turns into a wicked cough. Her chest x-ray shows she's got bronchitis, but it also shows something else: a vertebral fracture.

"How—and when—could that ever have happened?" she wonders.

Her doctor nods, explaining that many people experience vertebral fractures without knowing it. In fact, as many as two-thirds of all vertebral spine fractures may go unrecognized. The doctor orders a bone mineral density test, which confirms her suspicions that Helen's bone has thinned.

While educating Helen about the delicate state of her bones, the doctor goes through a list of dos and don'ts.

Tops on the list of don'ts: Avoid lifting bags in and out of overhead compartments on planes and trains. Also, avoid lugging those ubiquitous plastic bags from the store to your car using your fingers. It's too easy to snap a finger bone that way. Instead, ask for paper, not plastic, and get a good grip on the bottom of a properly filled bag.

Sound like odd tips? Get ready for the new world we face as we—and our bones—age.

Fractures: Affecting Men and Women Alike

Fracture risks increase greatly through the years, regardless of whether you're a man or a woman. About 1.5 million Americans will fracture bones due to osteoporosis every year, according to the National Osteoporosis Foundation. Here is how the numbers break down:

- 300,000 hip fractures
- 700,000 vertebral (spine) fractures
- 250,000 wrist fractures
- 300,000 fractures at other sites

About a third of these fracture patients—some 500,000 Americans—will require hospitalization. And many of those hospitalized patients will undergo costly surgery and rehabilitation.

Where Can Fractures Occur?

Hip Fractures. The World Health Organization has documented that broken hips are the most costly type of fracture and the most serious in terms of morbidity and mortality. Risks for these painful fractures are higher for women— 17 percent, versus 6 percent for men. In 2005, 293,000 Americans age 45 or older were admitted to U.S. hospitals with hip fractures, and osteoporosis was the cause of almost all of these serious fractures. These fractures threaten the patient's independence and life span. Approximately one in two women and one in four women over the age of 50 will have an osteoporosis-related fracture in their remaining lifetime. At least 20 percent of those who were ambulatory prior to their hip fracture require long-term care following the fracture, and only 15 percent of them will be able to walk unaided across a room six month after their fracture. My mother's fracture was followed by hip replacement surgery, blood transfusions, and a long hospitalization and rehabilitation, and although she lives independently, she still has difficulty with pain. Her small frame, positive family history, and height loss should have been clues that she had osteoporosis, and treatment could have prevented her hip fracture.

Many will die after their hip fractures, and the one-year mortality after a hip fracture is twice as high for men as for women. Women with a hip fracture are at a fourfold increased risk of a second one. A woman's risk of hip fracture is equal to her combined risk of breast, uterine, and ovarian cancer.

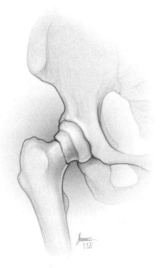

Hospital stays for a hip fracture can last as long as one month. Immobility due to hospitalization and recovery increases the risk of complications, including further bone loss. That may be one reason that having one hip fracture increases the risks of having another one.

Hip fractures usually involve a fracture of the "neck" of the femur, as illustrated here.

Just one-third of the individuals who suffer hip fractures regain their normal level of functioning. That means a nursing home—considered a fate worse than death by many an independent senior.

Spine Fractures. Vertebral fractures—compression, flattening, or crushing of the small bones in the spinal column—are a complicated matter. First of all, many vertebral fractures are silent, producing literally no symptoms at all.

Second, no universally accepted definition of *vertebral fracture* exists. So calculations of their incidence and healthcare costs vary, according to the definition used.

What is known is that 20 to 25 percent of postmenopausal Caucasian women have at least one deformed vertebra, and approximately 10 percent have a vertebral fracture severe enough to produce symptoms. Currently, the best estimate is that 30 to 50 percent of American women will suffer a spinal fracture during their lifetimes.

Like hip fractures, vertebral fractures increase both morbidity and mortality. Those who suffer a vertebral fracture have a 20 percent risk of suffering another one within the year. Multiple vertebral fractures can lead to the forward spinal curvature called kyphosis and a loss of height. Kyphosis, in turn, can trigger chronic back pain.

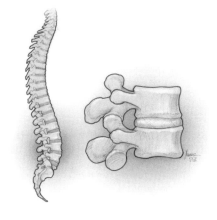

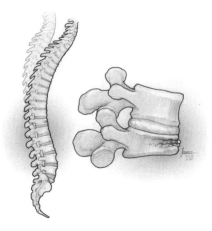

Vertebral or spine fractures involve compressions of the vertebrea, the bones of the spine as illustrated in the panel on the bottom.

The risk of other fractures also rises after a vertebral fracture. A history of spine fracture increases a woman's risk of hip fracture twofold. While spinal fractures aren't as deadly as

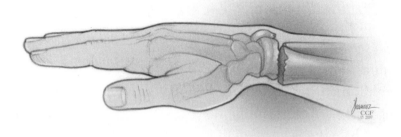

Wrist (forearm) fractures can involve both the radius and the ulna, two bones in the forearm.

hip fractures, they erode quality of life just the same, creating ever greater dependence on others.

Forearm Fractures. Fractures of the distal forearm (the bone near the wrist) are the next runner-up in terms of incidence among middle-aged and elderly Americans. Forearm fractures are usually caused by an attempt to break one's fall on the ice or stairs, as Kate, whom we met in chapter 2, experienced.

These fractures cause less morbidity and mortality than hip fractures, but they are painful, prompting tenderness, stiffness, and swelling in the hand. Forearm fractures can mean up to six weeks in a cast and surgery (or surgeries). They also increase the risks of other fractures in later life, but they do not impact mortality.

Falls: Facing Facts

As we age, our bones become more fragile, and our reflexes and vision aren't what they used to be. We just can't sidestep falls the way we once did.

Imagine yourself outside on a winter day. You hit a patch of ice your eye didn't detect.

The younger you would have started slipping and finessed the fall, maybe wobbling a bit. Looking a bit like a cartoon character, the only damage you'd feel would be that bruise to your ego.

Fast forward to you at age 58 or 65. You are busily doing errands and slip in a parking lot on a winter day, and you hit the ice. As you're going down, you brace your fall with your wrist—and crack! Your wrist snaps. But that's just the beginning. The doctor tells you that you've also fractured a vertebra. "You were just lucky you didn't break a hip," he

Facts About Falls

The U.S. surgeon general reported the following in 2004:

- One-third of individuals over age 65 fall each year; in half those cases, the person has fallen previously.

- One in ten falls in this age group results in serious injury, such as a hip fracture.

- Ninety percent of hip fractures are the result of falls.

- Among the elderly, falls account for 10 percent of visits to the emergency room and 6 percent of urgent hospitalizations.

- An elderly person with no risk factors has a 10 percent chance of falling each year.

- An elderly person with four or more risk factors has an 80 percent chance of falling each year.

says. Most patients who have wrist fractures are not tested for osteoporosis, and most are not treated.

After a certain age, we're at greater risk not only of falling but also of fracturing bones when we do fall. Low bone mass and osteoporosis are usually to blame.

Am I Actually More Likely to Fall as I Age?

Falling is rarely due to a single cause. Advancing age and increasing frailty are just two of the many factors affecting balance, gait, and coordination. That is why the American Geriatrics Society and the American Academy of Orthopaedic Surgeons Panel on Falls Prevention recommends annual health screenings and medication reviews for those prone to falls.

Falling is one of the prime reasons that the elderly lose their independence. Those who fall are more likely than others to fear another fall. Consciously or not, they restrict their activity. This adds to both perceived and actual frailty, as seniors hesitate to go out or to exercise.

How Do I Reduce My Risk of Falling?

A doctor can uncover risk factors that increase your chances of falling during your annual physical exam. These include the following:

- A history of falling
- The presence of arthritis
- Signs of depression
- Reports of dizziness

- The presence of chronic disease
- The need for home healthcare
- An acute illness

There are several options to help reduce your risk of falling, depending on the results of your exam.

Medications. The number and type of medications you take can predispose you to falls. That's why your doctor should periodically review all your medications and their side effects—including over-the-counter medicines for colds, etc.

Merely taking four or more medications increases risks of falling because the potential for problem drug interactions increases. As we age, our bodies metabolize medications more slowly, so smaller doses produce heightened effects. The result can be dizziness or lightheadedness.

Some medications can increase risks of falling because they impact blood pressure, cause dehydration, or affect balance (as sedatives and antidepressants do). Often, alternate medications can be substituted to manage the same medical problem—but with fewer side effects.

Vision. Annual eye exams are important to reduce risks of falling. Wearing glasses that don't properly correct vision is a risk factor for falls among seniors. Worsening eyesight due to glaucoma or cataracts also increases the likelihood of falls.

Footwear. Improper footwear is often to blame for falls. Most seniors are well aware that high heels increase the risks of falling. However, many are unaware that walking barefoot or in stocking feet at home increases the likelihood of falls. And home is where most seniors fall—typically by tripping but also by losing balance, feeling dizzy, or having the legs "give way."

A British Geriatrics Society report links fall-related hip fractures to potentially hazardous footwear. Wearing slippers, sandals, and indoor slip-ons without "fixation" (laces, buckles, straps, Velcro, or zippers) encourages shuffling, which can trigger tripping.

Soles that are too soft or too stiff are also linked to falls. The Centers for Disease Control recommends that seniors wear shoes with good support and thin, hard, nonslip soles. Shoes with more surface contacting the ground lessen the risks of falling. Shoes with deep treads are not recommended.

Fall-Proofing the Home. Fractures can occur whether we fall or not. Yet the importance of making our homes fall-proof cannot be overemphasized. Almost half of all falls happen at home, according to the Centers for Disease Control National Center for Injury Prevention and Control. (For seniors, "home" may mean a nursing home or long-term care facility.)

It's imperative to review living areas periodically to ensure that they are fall-proof. Do bathrooms and hallways have night-lights? Are tiles nonslip? Do throw rugs have nonskid backing? Can floors or stairways be cleared of clutter? Can the presence of a small pet cause a fall?

You can request a home hazard assessment by asking your primary doctor or geriatrics specialist to recommend an occupational therapist or a specialist in physical medicine and rehabilitation. Cleveland Clinic physical medicine and rehabilitation specialists offer a Falls Prevention Clinic specifically to help seniors and their family members reduce the likelihood of falls.

CDC Recommendations for Fall-Proofing Your Home

The CDC recommends the following steps for fall-proofing your home:

- Remove things you can trip over (such as papers, books, clothes, and shoes) from stairs and places where you walk.

- Remove small throw rugs or use double-sided tape to keep the rugs from slipping.

- Keep items you use often in cabinets you can reach easily without using a step stool.

- Have grab bars put in next to your toilet and in the tub or shower.

- Use nonslip mats in the bathtub and on shower floors.

- Improve the lighting in your home. As you get older, you need brighter lights to see well. Lamp shades or frosted bulbs can reduce glare.

- Have handrails and lights put in on all staircases.

Exercising. Lack of exercise increases the risks of falling, so an exercise program is an intrinsic part of a falls prevention strategy. Exercise will not only make seniors stronger and improve their balance; it will also make them feel more upbeat. Exercises that are most beneficial in falls prevention are those that blend muscle strengthening with balance retraining. Tai chi (sometimes called "meditation through movement") is an excellent example of this type of exercise.

The gentle Chinese discipline builds muscle strength and enhances flexibility through a series of slow, controlled, fluid movements. Ask your doctor if tai chi or another form of exercise might be beneficial for you or your loved one.

Leaning on Assistive Devices. Canes, walkers, and other assistive devices can help the frail elderly to maintain their balance. In nursing homes, bed alarms may also be used to alert staff when residents need help getting out of bed. Other devices include hip protectors that cushion the blow in case fragile seniors fall. Studies show that hip protectors can reduce hip fractures among the elderly who are in nursing homes or who require in-home assistance. However, hip protectors are ineffective on their own and must be part of a multipronged falls-prevention strategy.

Bone-Building Supplements and Medication. Vitamin D and calcium supplementation have been shown to reduce the risks of fractures due to falls. Medication that slows bone loss will not necessarily reduce fracture risks for those with low bone mass, but it may well stave off further bone loss.

A Good Social Network. When it comes to protecting the elderly who are still living on their own from falls, a strong family network and support system can't be beat. These two factors strongly correlate with a reduced risk of falling.

Chapter 9

The Future Is Now

In today's world, prevention and treatment for osteoporosis are changing rapidly, even daily. New delivery methods are being investigated for established therapies. New treatments are on the horizon, and some are available in clinical trials. Most primary care physicians, like Anne's below, and specialists will make sure they are informed of the latest study results and approved treatments.

Anne

Anne lives with multiple health problems that make managing her osteoporosis a challenge. She is a cancer survivor and had radiation therapy to her bones. Her esophagus has a narrowing, or stricture, that makes swallowing difficult. Yet Anne's numerous fractures indicate osteoporosis, which requires osteoporosis medication.

Unfortunately, her esophageal stricture rules out oral bisphosphonates, such as alendronate and risedronate, due to risks of irritation. Her susceptibility to nonvertebral hip, wrist, and other fractures means that she is not a candidate for raloxifene, the estrogen-like compound that has been demonstrated to protect only against spinal fractures. And her history of radiation therapy means she will not qualify for teriparatide, the bone-building, active form of parathyroid hormone.

You might think that Anne has run out of options. Fortunately, her doctor is aware of other possibilities.

So Anne's doctor orders lab work and checks her vitamin D levels. She determines that she is eligible for treatment with yearly IV zoledronic acid. She can come in just once a year and have the drug infused while sitting in a chair for 15 minutes. The medicine will go directly to her bones, bypassing her sensitive digestive system. She will, of course, need to continue her daily calcium and vitamin D supplements and maintain a consistent weight-bearing exercise program, but since her medication is given by a yearly IV route, it will not irritate her gastrointestinal tract.

IV Bisphosphonates

The FDA approval of some IV bisphosphonates for the treatment of osteoporosis has allowed a new route of administration for this well-established class of medications.

Research has reported that in three-year trials involving 7,700 postmenopausal women, yearly IV zoledronate reduced the risks of hip, spine, and nonvertebral fractures. It has also been shown to decrease the risk of subsequent fractures in patients who have already had an osteoporosis-related fracture and to increase the survival of those who have had a low-trauma hip fracture. Recent studies have shown it to be possibly more effective than some of the oral bisphosphonates in preventing bone loss in patients on steroids. It cannot be given to people with kidney failure or to those with abnormal calcium blood levels.

IV bisphosphonates also look promising for maintaining the increase in bone density that was gained with teriparatide treatment, which patients must stop taking the drug after two years of treatment.

The convenience of once-a-year IV delivery of bisphosphonates is highly appealing. Some studies show that only a minority of patients still take their osteoporosis medication after one or two years. Some people may not remember to take the pill at the same time each week or each month. Other people may find it inconvenient to swallow the pill on an empty stomach and then stay on their feet for 30 to 60 minutes while it is absorbed. Once-a-year IV bisphosphonate administration provides a treatment option for many who need bisphosphonate treatment but who are not otherwise able to take these medications.

Denosumab

Denosumab is an example of a new medication springing from intensive research. This medication has been submitted to the FDA for approval for the treatment of osteoporosis.

It is a fully human natural antibody that inhibits the molecule known as RANKL, which is important for osteoclast survival and development, and it then regulates bone resorption. Researchers reported that denosumab increased bone mineral density and decreased bone resorption in postmenopausal women with low bone mass.

Denosumab is injected beneath the skin at six-month intervals and in clinical trials it was shown to reduce significantly hip, spine and nonvertebral fractures in postmenopausal women. It has a positive effect on bone architecture, increasing bone density by 3.0 to 6.7 percent in the lower spine, by 1.9 to 3.6 percent in the hip, and by 0.4 to 1.3 percent in the forearm. Twelve months of treatment proved denosumab more effective than either the standard osteoporosis drug alendronate or a placebo.

Denosumab also shows promise in counteracting bone loss arising from conditions such as multiple myeloma and rheumatoid arthritis.

Sophisticated molecular studies will pave the way for other novel medications for osteoporosis. Such research may soon yield more effective means of increasing bone density, while decreasing fracture risks and side effects.

Other Avenues of Research

Research is ongoing on other fronts as well. While bone density tests continue to be the standard means of assessing bone health, we still seek improved ways to measure changes in bone architecture. Our goal is to understand further the nature of osteoporosis and osteopenia. Doing so will allow us to provide patients with better solutions in terms of preventing, treating, and reversing bone loss.

Staying in Touch

You and your doctor are partners in managing your bone health. More and more physicians are reviewing their treatment plans for osteoporosis as advances are reported in prevention, testing, and treatment. I hope that you will stay in close contact with your own doctor to ensure that you stay abreast of the rapid changes occurring in our field.

Conclusion

L iving with severe osteoporosis can be devastating. It can mean that actions as seemingly nontraumatic as picking up a grandchild, leaning over to pick up a golf ball, or just coughing can result in broken bones. The resultant fractures of the ribs, spine, or hip could lead to months of severe pain, surgery, loss of independence, or even death. Osteoporosis is not just a cosmetic condition that we strive to avoid so that we can maintain posture. And osteoporosis is not just an inevitable consequence of aging. Jack's fracture on the golf course could have been avoided if knowledge about male osteoporosis had led to him getting a bone density test earlier and his osteoporosis had been treated before the fracture. My mother's hip fracture after falling in a bank on a slushy day in February could have been avoided if her osteoporosis had been detected earlier. And my grandmother's painful vertebral compression fracture could have been prevented if she had been treated at the time of her wrist fracture ten years earlier.

With appropriate attention to bone health in childhood, adolescence, and young adulthood, strong bones can be built that will help sustain the skeleton into older age. And when adults face the loss of bone mass in their 50s and 60s, treatments are available to maintain and build bone. For people who do have severe osteoporosis, many treatments can increase bone mass and prevent the occurrence of subsequent fractures. I have many patients who are now living active lives, doing activities that had previously resulted in fractures. It is so gratifying to hear of their babysitting their grandchildren, their travels, and their athletic activities after treatment for their osteoporosis was underway.

Yet we still have so many challenges. Most people with osteoporosis are still not diagnosed or treated. Even the majority of people with fractures from osteoporosis are not diagnosed with the disease. Most individuals with significant risk factors for bone loss and fractures do not know that they are at risk for osteoporosis. Many people on treatment abandon their medication due to side effects or misleading media reports about possible toxicities. Simple measures like fall prevention are not emphasized in most medical settings. Support for new scientific discoveries in the area of metabolic bone research is inadequate. And lack of sufficient insurance coverage of bone density testing threatens patient access to this important test.

I hope that you have learned some of the key facts about bone health as you read this book. And I hope that you are inspired to learn more, share information with your friends and family, and be an advocate for the prevention and treatment of osteoporosis. If we are truly effective in focusing on bone health in childhood and young adulthood, we might be able to prevent this disease in many cases. New, exciting treatments on the horizon will improve the future for patients with osteoporosis. The future will be brighter as bone wellness becomes a priority for us all.

With wishes for your future bone health!

Abby Abelson, MD

Appendix 1

Web Resource Guide for Information on Osteoporosis

Knowing more about osteoporosis can make you a smarter healthcare consumer. Check out the following organizations and their websites for reliable information on health. Online research is a great starting point. But remember to check with your physician for a detailed and personalized prevention plan.

Cleveland Clinic Center for Consumer Health Information
www.clevelandclinic.org/health/

9500 Euclid Avenue
Cleveland, OH 44195
866-594-2276

Search for *osteoporosis* at this health information resource, and you'll discover a variety of detailed information on everything from basic osteoporosis facts to hip fractures in the elderly, osteoporosis and men, medications for and prevention of osteoporosis during menopause, and more.

National Osteoporosis Foundation (NOF)

www.nof.org

1232 22nd Street NW
Washington, DC 20037-1202
800-231-4222 or (202) 223-2226

This leading volunteer organization is solely dedicated to osteoporosis and bone health, focusing on awareness, education, and advocacy. Check out the latest information on calcium, bone health, and many other related topics. On the site, you can find a link to *The 2004 Surgeon General's Report on Bone Health and Osteoporosis.*

The National Institutes of Health (NIH) Osteoporosis and Related Bone Diseases— National Resource Center

www.niams.nih.gov/Health_Info/Bone/

2 AMS Circle
Bethesda, MD 20892-3676
800-624-BONE (800-624-2663) or (202) 466-4315

This center provides a wealth of information for patients and professionals on metabolic bone diseases, including osteoporosis, Paget's disease, hyperparathyroidism, and osteogenesis imperfecta, from the National Institutes of Health and the Department of Health and Human Services.

The National Institutes of Health (NIH) National Institute of Arthritis and Musculoskeletal and Skin Diseases

www.niams.nih.gov

Office of Communications and Public Liaison
National Institutes of Health
Bldg. 31, Room 4C02
31 Center Drive—MSC 2350
Bethesda, MD 20892-2350
(301) 496-8190

This branch of the National Institutes of Health supports research into the causes of musculoskeletal and skin diseases, including osteoporosis.

Powerful Bones, Powerful Girls: The National Bone Health Campaign

www.girlshealth.gov/bones/

1090 Vermont Ave, Third Floor
Washington, DC 20005
(202) 842-3600 x253
powerfulbones@hhs.gov

This colorful, animated website offers educational activities that encourage girls to take charge of their bone health.

CDC's Healthy Communities Program

www.cdc.gov/healthycommunitiesprogram/

Centers for Disease Control and Prevention
4770 Buford Highway NE
Mailstop K-93
Atlanta, GA 30341-3717
(770) 488-6452
cdcinfo@cdc.gov

This national, multilevel chronic disease prevention program works to reduce chronic diseases and attain health equity through training, mentorship, dissemination of effective models, and investments in communities that jump-start local change.

VERB Youth Media Campaign

www.cdc.gov/youthcampaign/

Division of Adolescent and School Health
4770 Buford Highway NE
MS K-29
Atlanta, GA 30341-3724
800-CDC-INFO (800-232-4636)
cdcinfo@cdc.gov

A national multicultural and social campaign, VERB encourages youths ages 9 to 13 ("tweens") to be physically active daily. It is coordinated by the Centers for Disease Control and Prevention.

American Dietetic Association

www.eatright.org

120 South Riverside Plaza, Suite 2000
Chicago, IL 60606-6995
800-877-1600

The largest organization of food and nutrition professionals, the American Dietetic Association promotes health, nutrition, and well-being. This helpful website offers easy-to-read information about nutrition and healthy eating habits and includes information on calcium-rich foods.

An excerpt from

The Cleveland Clinic Guide to

MENOPAUSE

By Holly L. Thacker, MD

Now available in
The Cleveland Clinic Guide Series

Symptoms
of Menopause

When some women approach midlife, they suddenly find themselves lost in an avalanche of debilitating symptoms that daily threaten their quality of life. Depression, anxiety, sleep loss—you name it. Menopause barrels into their lives like a runaway truck, damaging appearance, mood, sex life, and sense of self-worth. That's Kathy's predicament, and maybe it's yours, too.

Kathy

Everything in my life was falling into place like a Kodak moment. My two beautiful daughters announced their engagements, and our family—always so close—felt complete. We celebrated with gatherings whenever possible. My career allowed me more freedom to pursue hobbies I had put on hold for years, especially gardening, which I love. My husband and I even planned a postwedding cruise, anticipating the need for a break after a hectic year. The vacation would be a second honeymoon for us.

Our album of pictures from that year shows photographs of me smiling—beaming, even. Picture-perfect. I don't know how I held it together. Many days I didn't.

"Kathy just isn't Kathy," my sisters confided to each other. They were right. My periods had stopped, and my body had abruptly changed. My panic attacks were unpredictable and uncontrollable. Frighteningly, at night, a racing heartbeat shook my whole body. My legs and arms would go numb as I imagined myself in a wheelchair, my life crashing down around me. I headed to more than one emergency room and consulted several doctors.

Of course, my husband, Bill, loved me, comforted me, and held me. He knew I wasn't getting better, and neither of us could pretend differently.

I couldn't sleep, which made everything worse. I was still smiling and trying to hold it together for my daughters on the outside, but I was falling apart on the inside. How could a mother and wife be so distressed and feel so desperate during what was supposed to be a happy time?

I finally visited a physician who specialized in women's health. After conducting a complete physical exam, gyne-cological exam, hormonal assessment, and series of tests, she determined that my symptoms were associated with hormone fluctuations, the onset of menopause, and panic disorder, all very treatable conditions.

"You're kidding!" I said to her. Unbelievable. These symp-toms were not the classic hot flashes I'd had heard about.

On a scale of one to ten for menopause symptoms, Kathy's case pushes the limit. Her situation is somewhat unusual, although no woman's experience while her reproductive system winds down could be classified as "normal." This goes back to my point that every woman is different; one woman may breeze through menopause, not realizing that she is officially "in menopause" until she counts off twelve menstruation-free months. Ta-da—a seamless transition. Her life is barely affected by "the change." Another may suffer the way Kathy did—until she received proper treatment, that is.

Menopause Is Natural

During this time, it's important to remember that *menopause is a natural part of aging. It is not a disease.* However, just as with menstruation and childbirth, an educated assessment and some medical attention may be necessary.

Many of my patients nearing their early 50s regard the years leading up to menopause (called perimenopause) as a living hell. But they don't have to be.

If your symptoms make you feel like the shell of the person you were just months ago, you're probably wondering "Why me?" The answer to this question is multifaceted. First, we must understand what happens inside a woman's body during the onset of menopause. Because menopause varies with every woman, knowledge is the best tool for maintaining a positive attitude.

The Inside Story

A woman's life can be divided into three hormonal phases, comparable to the acts in a play:

- Reproduction
- Menopause
- Postmenopause

The pituitary gland in the brain is the "director," telling the body how much of certain hormones to make during each of the three phases. Furthermore, current medical thinking recognizes that what most people refer to as "menopause" is actually a process involving three stages: perimenopause, menopause, and postmenopause.

What Is Perimenopause?

During this period, ovarian function becomes erratic. A woman may detect physical signs, such as hot flashes and irregular periods. Perimenopause usually begins sometime in a woman's 40s and lasts a full year after the final menstrual period.

What Is Menopause?

This is the time when the ovaries stop releasing eggs and a woman no longer has periods. Menopause usually occurs between the ages of 45 and 55. A general indication of menopause is cessation of periods for twelve consecutive months. The average age for women to experience menopause in this country is 51.3 years.

• • • Fast Fact • • •

The term *menopause* comes from the Greek *meno,* meaning month, and *pausis,* a pause or stop.

• • •

What Is Postmenopause?

The postmenopausal time frame is divided into early postmenopause—the first five years since the last menstrual period—and late postmenopause—five years and beyond. The early postmenopausal phase is the most critical in terms of symptoms and bone loss and is generally the time frame that hormone therapy is initiated if indicated. You can not base medical decisions on age alone; a 55-year-old woman could be ten years past menopause in the late postmenopausal phase, she could still be menstruating and be premenopausal, or she could be starting to skip menses and be perimenopausal or in the "menopause transition."

What's Causing All of This Change?

Our levels of estrogen, testosterone, and progesterone, the main characters in our cast of hormones, fluctuate throughout our lives. This up-and-down process sometimes produces happy endings. At other times, hormone imbalance creates conflict. And the plot thickens.

Estrogen. Estrogen is the term for a class of female sex hormones secreted by the ovaries. The three major kinds of estrogens are estriol, estradiol, and estrone.

Estrogen influences the development and maintenance of typical female sex characteristics, such as increased body fat in hips and thighs and smoother skin (compared to men). Estrogen also influences the female reproductive system in many ways, including preparing the body for reproduction.

Progesterone. Progesterone is a steroid hormone that prepares the uterus for pregnancy, maintains pregnancy, and promotes development of the mammary glands. The main sources of progesterone are the corpus luteum (formed after ovulation in the ovary) and the placenta.

The term *progestogens* encompasses both progestins (synthetic versions of the hormone) and progesterone itself.

Testosterone. Testosterone affects sex-related features and development. In men, it is produced in large amounts by the testicles. In both men and women, testosterone is also produced in small amounts by the adrenal glands and, in women, by the ovaries.

Estrogen Plays the Lead. Let's focus for a minute on the key hormone that signals menopause onset—our leading lady, estrogen. Before a woman goes into menopause, more than 90 percent of her estrogen is made by the ovaries. (Organs that make smaller amounts include the adrenal glands, the liver, and kidneys.)

Estrogen regulates your monthly cycles of ovulation and menstruation. It also plays a role in your psychological well-being, which covers your mood, sleep, and sex drive; your urinary tract; your skin and vaginal tissues; and your bones and heart. In addition, estrogen is involved in your blood-vessel tone and the health of your gums, teeth, and eyes.

Historically, estrogen has been "typecast" as the girls-only hormone, regarded for its role in women's reproductive functions. It is applauded for helping to bring babies into the world and for creating women's attractive hourglass figures—sometimes it's blamed when those figures keep us from fitting into our favorite jeans.

Estrogen is all woman. And, like women, estrogen has a brainy side.

Estrogen affects the brain's blood flow. It can boost verbal memory (testosterone supports spatial memory) and improve the way the brain processes information. Estrogen can also affect mood. For example, decreased estrogen levels can affect serotonin levels, which in turn can spark anxiety and/or depression. This explains why a woman with no medical history of depression may go through a bout just as she enters menopause.

• • • *Fast Fact* • • •

It's ironic that the average 55-year-old man may have a higher estrogen level than the average 55-year-old woman. That is because men usually enjoy steady testosterone production as they age, and testosterone is regularly converted into small amounts of estradiol/estrogen. But a woman suffers from decreased estrogen production as she enters menopause. A woman who loses her ovaries or her eggs no longer has a constant source of estradiol production.

• • •

Short-term Symptoms

When your ovaries stop making estrogen, you go into menopause, and your periods end. For all intents and purposes, estrogen has left the stage.

But as we've just seen, estrogen isn't involved only in your reproductive system. Other body systems are affected by estrogen levels, too, so it's easy to understand why menopause gets its tentacles into so many areas of physical, mental, and emotional function.

Unfortunately, we usually don't realize how important estrogen is to maintaining physical and mental balance until we are running on empty. Then, strange symptoms often suggest that something different is going on in the body.

Here's a list of common menopausal symptoms:

- **Hot flashes.** Sudden sensations of heat that spread from the chest to head, often followed by sweating and cold shivering. A hot flush is not the flash but the redness that suffuses the neck and face. (See chapter 7 for more about hot flashes.)

- **Night sweats.** Hot flashes that occur during sleep and cause perspiration.

- **Difficulty sleeping.** Often related to hot flashes and night sweats.

- **Vaginal changes.** These include dryness and increased vulnerability to bladder infections.

- **Sex drive.** Mood changes can affect a woman's interest in sex, as can vaginal dryness, making sex more uncomfortable.

- **Mood changes.** These can include irritability, anxiety, and mood swings.

- **Skin changes.** These include dryness, itching, and loss of elasticity.

- **Headaches/migraines.** These may be worsened by hormone fluctuations, although migraines usually get better after menopause. (For more information on migraines, see appendix 3.)

- **Heart palpitations.** These can be manifestations of symptoms (such as hot flashes) in the autonomic system (the nerves and muscles that cause the blood vessels to constrict or dilate), but any heart symptom needs to be checked out by a doctor before being attributed to menopause.

- **Hair.** Increased facial hair or thinning hair on the head can be due to lack of estrogen and/or increased sensitivity to remaining testosterone.

- **Memory loss/poor concentration.** Forgetfulness or reduced ability to think clearly can be related to hormone fluxes, lack of sleep, increased stressors, undiagnosed medical problems, vitamin deficiencies, or depression.

Age-related Changes

For all women, aging and menopause go hand in hand—so, naturally, the estrogen loss of menopause is linked to a number of health problems that are considered common signs of aging. After menopause, women are more likely to suffer from the following:

- **Changes in bladder function.** These can be age related, or they can result from genetic predisposition, childbearing trauma, or weight gain. (Bladder function can become more overactive with the loss of estrogen.)

- **Poor brain function.** This includes an increased risk of Alzheimer's disease associated with advanced age.

- **Loss of skin elasticity.** This results in increased wrinkling.

- **Decreased muscle tone and bone loss.**

- **Some changes in vision.**

- **Weight fluctuation and slower metabolism.**

Some women feel defeated when they confront these issues. We can't stop the clock, after all. But you can control many of these problems with relative ease by eating well, exercising regularly, protecting the skin from sun damage, taking the right vitamins and supplements, and staying actively involved in life as you work with your physician to design a personalized regimen. (We'll talk more about age versus hormones in chapter 3.)

Long-term Problems

There are long-term risks that women inherit with age and menopause. Heart disease and osteoporosis are two of the most serious. The heart and bones can suffer tremendously from estrogen deficiency, making it especially important to take measures to reduce cholesterol, lower blood pressure, refrain from smoking, and maintain bone mass.

Fortunately, lifestyle choices can modify these risks. We will discuss these and other ways to reduce these risks throughout this book.

Are We There Yet?

Estrogen doesn't usually vanish from your body all at once, without warning.

Decline in estrogen starts during perimenopause, the phase before full-blown menopause. During perimenopause, hormones begin to fluctuate, periods may occur at unpredictable intervals, and bleeding may be quite heavy and periodically hormone levels can surge.

Perimenopause usually begins in a woman's 40s, sometimes lasting as long as eight to ten years. This does *not* mean that over this entire period you will notice signs of the onset of menopause. It simply means that your ovaries are winding down their ovulatory function. In fact, you may not recognize any of the short-term symptoms we just discussed until you reach the last few years of perimenopause, when estrogen production drops more dramatically and more quickly.

Perimenopause lasts until menopause, when the ovaries stop releasing eggs completely.

How Can I Tell That I've Reached Menopause?

When a woman stops having her menstrual period and hasn't had one at all for twelve months, she is medically defined as menopausal. (We'll talk more about breakthrough or abnormal bleeding in chapter 13.)

How old you are when you experience menopause is related to the number of eggs in your ovaries, which is determined by a genetic component. If the women in your family generally go into menopause in their early 40s, chances are that you'll experience an early menopause, too.

Your lifestyle and medical history also can affect the age you'll be when you go into menopause. For example, smokers and women with chronic illness are more likely to experience early onset.

In certain cases, women may enter menopause without knowing it or can even experience induced menopause.

Can I Be Tested for Menopause?

Everyone wants a "menopause test," something that will predict when menopause will actually happen, but testing for menopause is a bit trickier than checking body temperature or diagnosing strep throat.

Red Flag

If a woman is over 50 years old, has gone even six months without a period (an indication of the onset of menopause), and then bleeds or spots, she should see a doctor within that month.

This kind of postmenopausal bleeding is often caused by treatable and relatively benign conditions. But in some cases—perhaps up to 5 percent—postmenopausal bleeding can indicate uterine cancer or a precursor, such as hyperplasia (an abnormal increase in cells).

If you do experience such bleeds or spots, you should get a Pap smear, pelvic exam, special saline-infusion sonogram (SIS), and an endometrial sampling, in which the doctor takes a biopsy, or small sampling, of the endometrium (the lining of the uterus) to examine.

For more on abnormal bleeding and what to do about it, see chapter 13.

The best way to confirm menopause is by analyzing symptoms associated with estrogen deficiency and performing a thorough history and physical exam, including the following:

- **Determination of menstrual patterns.** These include your age, menstrual history, and the number of months that you have missed your period, as well as the appearance of such classic symptoms as hot flashes.

- **Assessment of vaginal tissues.** The major indicator of menopause is the condition of the vaginal tissues, which are the body tissues most sensitive to estrogen loss. Normally, the vagina is thick, plush, and pink. In estrogen-deficient women, the vagina is thin, pale, flat, and dry. It also becomes more alkaline. If the vaginal tissue is really thin, it may appear red and can tear and bleed easily.

- **Measuring bone density and bone tissue.** Bone is sensitive to the levels of estrogen and other hormone levels, and it may show density loss when estrogen production decreases over time.

Still, many patients insist on black-and-white test results, and many physicians perform lab tests that, while offering a momentary snapshot of the various hormone levels, are not really at all helpful in diagnosing or predicting menopause.

The following tests are *not* accurate ways of confirming menopause and do *not* paint a picture of total body estrogen:

- **pH test.** When estrogen levels fall, pH levels in vaginal tissue increase. Your doctor can measure the pH levels in your vagina with simple pH paper in the office, but this is not a foolproof confirmation of menopause because some vaginal infections also cause vaginal pH levels to rise.

- **Saliva tests.** Saliva contains a fraction of the hormones that are in the bloodstream. Most salivary tests are a waste of money and are not a valid way to measure levels of progesterone, or estradiol (a potent type of estrogen), and testosterone. And even when we do know a woman's level of estradiol, we cannot predict when she will run out of eggs and, therefore, lose most of her estrogen production. In addition, cigarette smoke, certain foods, hormone therapy or hormonal contraception, and environmental stressors can affect the results of saliva tests.

- **Urinary tests.** Urine tests promising to give indications of menopause onset can be purchased without a prescription for home use. These measure pituitary gonadotrophins, which are typically elevated in menopause. Again, these are not always reliable because these levels begin to elevate during the years before menopause, so it could be as long as ten years later when menopause begins. Be aware that, even with elevated urine-test results, if you haven't gone twelve months without a period, you could still be premenopausal or perimenopausal, and you're still at risk for pregnancy.

- **Follicle-stimulating hormone (FSH) test.** FSH tests measure blood levels of FSH. FSH rises each month to encourage follicles in the ovaries to release eggs, causing a menstrual period. A high FSH level may indicate that your body is working hard to release eggs and may not be unsuccessful. Depending on how high the levels are, this may indicate perimenopause or menopause. But FSH levels fluctuate considerably from one minute to the next, thus making them unreliable indicators of menopause. The test is usually ordered within the first three days of the period (when the levels should be at lower levels) and can be used during infertility evaluations to assess ovarian reserve.

Many doctors simply order these tests to satisfy women who demand a "menopause test," but they are neither predictive nor definitive.

Are Menopause- and Estrogen-related Tests Reliable?

Ultimately, body fluid (blood, saliva, and urine) tests are not the most accurate ways to measure estrogen levels in women. Metabolism is complex where estrogen is concerned. A woman may have a low level of estrogen in the blood but high levels in certain body tissues. What's in your bloodstream or saliva is not as important as what's in such body tissues as the brain, breasts, bones, or reproductive and urinary system.

Alone, these tests are not reliable indicators of menopause. However, paired with a clinical evaluation, bone density test, and thorough physical examination, they can serve as supporting evidence. Persistently elevated FSH levels usually imply impending menopause.

• • • *Fast Fact* • • •

Premature menopause occurs in less than 1 percent of women under the age of 40. Reasons can range from autoimmune conditions to fragile X syndrome to chemotherapy treatment.

• • •

How Does Birth Control Affect Menopause?

In addition to its contraceptive uses, I sometimes prescribe the pill to alleviate symptoms during perimenopause. But if you are taking the pill, your periods won't tell you whether you're officially in menopause or not. (You still get periods when you're on the pill, even if your body wouldn't naturally menstruate.) So how do you know?

The only way to tell is to go off the pill. But keep in mind that the timing of such an experiment is up to you. If you're dealing with several heavy stressors in your life, it may not be the right time to experiment with your hormone levels.

For example, take Valerie.

Valerie

Valerie was a fifty-two-year-old patient of mine who asked me if I thought she should stop taking the pill. She didn't need the prescription for contraceptive purposes any more, since her husband had a vasectomy. However, she was finishing her master's degree and juggling a demanding career while caring for her ailing and elderly mother.

I asked her to consider whether this was really the best time to introduce another potential stress into her life. She decided to wait until she had earned her degree.

What Is Hormonal Contraception?

Today, birth control comes in a variety of forms collectively known as "hormonal contraception," or HC. HC includes the pill, the patch, the vaginal ring, uterine devices, and subdermal (under-the-skin) implants.

Of course, Valerie might have gone off the pill and felt just fine. But it was equally possible that once she did so, her hormones would have proceeded to rage out of control or precipitously drop to very low levels.

Here's the bottom line: If you're on the pill and don't smoke, and have normal blood pressure and overall good health, it's usually safe to continue taking the pill until you reach age 55. And it's fine to pick a time when life is not taking you for a spin to test how you feel when you're not taking hormones.

During this time, I always talk with my patients about symptoms of menopause so they understand what to expect. Some of them go off the pill, never get another period, and suffer few if any symptoms. Others crash into menopause with severe side effects.

If a woman comes off the pill and ends up having difficult symptoms, I may put her back on it if she still needs contraception. Or I'll prescribe hormone therapy. I try again later to take her off the pill.

• • • *Fast Fact* • • •

Estrogen therapy is not a risky solution to
menopausal symptoms for most women who
have had hysterectomies.

• • •

Hysterectomy and Hormone Therapy

Women who have had hysterectomies do not have menstrual periods, but they can still produce hormones (estrogen) if one or both ovaries are intact. In a woman who has had a hysterectomy but still has her ovaries, when her estrogen levels fall, she may experience symptoms of menopause just like any other woman.

Sometimes women who have had hysterectomies begin menopause a few years earlier because of disturbance to this sensitive reproductive area.

Women who have both the uterus and ovaries removed during a hysterectomy are likely to experience the immediate onset of menopausal symptoms because their bodies no longer produce estrogen. (No ovaries, no estrogen.) This type of menopause is known as surgical or induced menopause, and it tends to be more severe.

Many women who have had hysterectomies ease into menopause without a problem. Without a uterus, most of these women no longer experience monthly bleeding or pain, and they generally enjoy fulfilling sex lives. But there are no absolutes.

One of every six to ten women whose ovaries were removed during a hysterectomy is thrown into a tailspin during menopause. Not only are her hormones out of balance, her body may be depleted of estrogen and testosterone. Hysterectomy surgery can cause a woman to lose most or all of her estrogen and as much as 25 to 50 percent of her testosterone sources.

For most women in this situation, hormone therapy is an effective treatment choice for the alleviation of severe menopausal symptoms. And there are many different ways to take HT, including pills, creams, gels, vaginal rings, and patches.

When physicians deny women in this condition the opportunity to take hormone therapy, it's like telling a woman who needs shoes that she should be able to get along with slippers or boots, or just go barefoot.

Is Menopause Easier With or Without Ovaries?

A hysterectomy is a major surgery to remove a woman's uterus, often performed to treat a health issue. The procedure may also include removal of other reproductive organs, including one or both ovaries, the fallopian tubes, and the cervix.

I advise my patients to keep their ovaries until at least age 65 unless there is good reason to remove them, such as cancer or the presence of one of the mutations of the breast cancer gene (BRCA genes), which indicates high risk for breast and ovarian cancer.

When women are shut out of proven options like hormone therapy, we lose our freedom of choice and the ability to decide which solution is best for us.

You need a doctor who is knowledgeable about the women's health field and who presents all the options. Not all family physicians and OB-GYNs keep up with the latest studies on hormone therapy. Doctors should know that estrogen therapy is not a risky solution for most women with hysterectomies. However, even medical professionals can be influenced by the media.

If you've had your ovaries removed during hysterectomy, be sure that your doctor is familiar with all the therapy options. There's no reason for you to suffer.

Index

About the Author

Abby Abelson, MD, is the Interim Chair of the Department of Rheumatic and Immunologic Diseases of the Orthopaedic and Rheumatology Institute at Cleveland Clinic. She is also the Director of Education of the Center for Osteoporosis and Metabolic Bones Disease and the Education Program Director for the Department of Rheumatic and Immunologic Diseases of Cleveland Clinic. She is also a Basic Science Course Director and a Physician Advisor in the Cleveland Clinic Lerner College of Medicine.

She is a graduate of Case Western Reserve University School of Medicine where she was elected to the Alpha Omega Alpha medical honor society and was given the Alice Paige Cleveland Award for "Outstanding Leadership Qualities."

She has presented multiple CME national conferences on the subject of osteoporosis and other metabolic bone diseases including the National Osteoporosis Foundation, the American Society of Reproductive Medicine, the American College of Obstetrics and Gynecology, and the American College of Physicians. She has presented on glucocorticoid osteoporosis at the Annual Review course of the Cleveland Review of Rheumatic Disease.

In addition to *The Cleveland Clinic Guide to Osteoporosis,* she authored the chapters "Preservation of Bone Density in Postmenopausal Women" and "Women at Risk: The Premenopausal Years" in *The Female Patient.* She also co-authored the chapter on "Osteoporosis Treatment" in *Hochberg's Rheumatology.* She acted as Rheumatology Editor and wrote chapters for *Current Clinical Medicine: 2009.* She also authored the chapter "Osteoarthritis" in *Women's Health in Primary Care.*

She is a member and past Chair of the Medical and Scientific Committee and is a member of the Board of the Northeast Ohio Arthritis Foundation. In 2001 and 2005, she was awarded volunteer leadership awards by that organization.

She has been named in "Best Doctors in America" from 1998 to 2009 and is listed in the Center for the Study of Services' *Guide to Top Doctors.*

About Cleveland Clinic

Cleveland Clinic, located in Cleveland, Ohio, is a not-for-profit multispecialty academic medical center that integrates clinical and hospital care with research and education.

Cleveland Clinic was founded in 1921 by four renowned physicians with a vision of providing outstanding patient care based upon the principles of cooperation, compassion, and innovation. *U.S. News & World Report* consistently names Cleveland Clinic as one of the nation's best hospitals in its annual "America's Best Hospitals" survey. Approximately 1,800 full-time salaried physicians and researchers at Cleveland Clinic and Cleveland Clinic Florida represent more than 100 medical specialties and subspecialties. In 2007, there were 3.5 million outpatient visits to Cleveland Clinic and 50,455 hospital admissions. Patients came for treatment from every state and from more than 80 countries. Cleveland Clinic's website address is *www.clevelandclinic.org.*